Holding
Tight,
Letting
Go

SARAH HUGHES

Holding Tight, Letting Go

MY LIFE, DEATH AND ALL THE MADNESS IN BETWEEN

BLINK
bringing you closer

First published in the UK by Blink Publishing
An imprint of Bonnier Books UK
4th Floor, Victoria House,
Bloomsbury Square,
London, WC1B 4DA

Owned by Bonnier Books
Sveavägen 56, Stockholm, Sweden

facebook.com/blinkpublishing
twitter.com/blinkpublishing

Hardback – 9781788705080
Ebook – 9781788705097
Audiobook - 9781788705103

A CIP catalogue of this book is available from the British Library.

Designed by Envy Design Ltd

Printed and bound in Great Britain by Clays Ltd, Elcograf S.p.A

1 3 5 7 9 10 8 6 4 2

Blink Publishing is an imprint of Bonnier Books UK
www.bonnierbooks.co.uk

Contents

Introduction
by Harriet Tyce

IF YOU'RE LUCKY, THERE'S A FRIEND YOU MAKE WHO BECOMES INTEGRAL TO YOUR WHOLE LIFE. Sarah was that friend for me. I'd been at the same Edinburgh school from Primary 1 through the tortures of middle school, resigning myself to its monochrome ways and bizarre domination by those girls who excelled at hockey, when Sarah burst in at the start of senior school, lighting the place up with colour and music I'd never heard of, introducing me to whole new worlds.

I thought the operettas of Gilbert and Sullivan counted as pop music. She played me Pink Floyd and the Cure. I was obsessed with getting top marks for vocabulary tests; she read Virginia Andrews and showed me the infamous goldfish scene in Shirley Conran's *Lace*. She wasn't just cool, though. She was kind, too. That year that everyone gave me Body Shop shampoo for greasy hair – 13 is the cruellest age – Sarah gave me Rimmel eyeshadow, greys and the softest pink, refraining from comment on my acne and slick locks.

As we turned 14, 15, we were on the cusp of life, and Sarah was brimming over with it. We met boys in Princes Street Gardens, drank vodka with them in the graveyard near the West End. We'd talk long through the day and then later into the evening, her phone number still emblazoned on my memory, 447 1443. One Easter holiday, I made a reverse-charge call to her house from the Highlands where I was staying – the bill for that call was £50, a lot of money for a call at any time, but especially in 1988. There was always something to talk about; the words never ran out.

Later, when she went to boarding school, the words were written. I still have those letters;

rereading them now transports me straight back to those heady days of boys and smoking, discos and balls. We gossiped, we bitched. If she had nothing to say, stuck in the midst of the rolling hills of Surrey as she was, she made stories up, elaborate fantasies as to why she'd forgotten my birthday or what she'd do to the friends who were being slower to write. She came up with a particularly brilliant list of potential deaths for someone who was being mean to me – we'd read *Papillon* recently, and red ants played a large role. *You don't understand how much it means to get a letter*, she said. But when it was a letter from her, I knew exactly how much it meant.

University followed, the letters still passing between us from one end of the country to the other. She had a boyfriend, a boy with green eyes. She'd made friends with the cool kids who'd terrified me at my sixth form – and through her they became less terrifying if not less cool, though of course none was cooler than Sarah. We reconnected in holidays, drinking the pubs of Edinburgh dry; indie discos, Nirvana, a pack of Marlboro Reds never far out of reach. A night out with Sarah was living, exactly as you'd want it to be.

Our twenties passed. Letters were fading, emails just beginning. Sarah was in New York; I in London. Our paths crossed, crossed again, a reconnection proper happening in 1999. I was getting married; she'd broken up with the boy with green eyes. My wedding was soon after that break up and she appeared dressed as a Sicilian widow, her black hat with its black veil a gift from her brother from Amsterdam. I'd later wear a hat like it at her funeral. It was the worst social occasion of her life, she told me a couple of years ago, but she may have been exaggerating for effect. Sarah could be like that, sometimes. Though never with the important stuff.

A job at the *Manchester Evening News* followed. We'd visit her one-bed flat in Salford, each weekend a different party with new friends or meal in a new restaurant. I'm not sure she ever cooked a meal in the tiny kitchen – it would have breached most food hygiene rules if she had. Cleaning was never Sarah's strong point, time wasted when she could be writing or reading. Her book recommendations were always on point but I remember the ones from those years particularly – George R. R. Martin, a fantasy writer I might enjoy, back before the series was even a twinkle in HBO's eye.

Back in London, she worked at the *Guardian* and we'd meet at the Coach and Horses in Clerkenwell, sinking whiskies late into the night. It was there she told me she had a new boyfriend, Kris. Without delay she introduced him to her friends; it was clear to us that she'd met the love of her life. They met via their support of their beloved Tottenham Hotspur but their connection went far beyond football. They were truly compatible in every way. No one could make more of a drama out of a minor crisis than Sarah, her temper snapping at the smallest of hiccups, but Kris was impervious to her rage, laughing at its excess and bringing a counterweight of calm that allowed her to flourish.

She called to tell me they had become engaged and, drunk, I raced across London in a taxi, certain that they could ask for no better celebration than to have me appear, clutching a bottle of champagne. Their wedding was riotous, a perfect celebration wholly befitting of them, before they moved to New York, almost immediately having their daughter Ruby in 2007 (only three months before my daughter was born) and their son Oisín in 2009. These were the happiest days of their lives, the best of times.

Or rather, they should have been. Clouds were beginning to gather. As Sarah lays out in her chapters here, in 2011 they lost their unborn daughter Iris at 36 weeks' pregnancy in a tragic stillbirth. Ruby and Oisín were so small, still, their needs so paramount, that family and friends went over to help, staying with Sarah and Kris in the rawness of their early grief. Sarah was recovering physically, too, from the caesarean section that had been necessary to deliver Iris.

You might think it would have been a visit of unmitigated sadness but this was the first intimation I had of the way that Sarah and Kris could live with resilience in times of the greatest sadness. Even at that time, I remember we managed to laugh on occasion. I had just started to write and I shared some of the work with Sarah, who was even then able to give time and energy to discuss what I was doing. Bring books from Heathrow, she had asked, keen to take refuge in the latest bonkbusters available in airport exclusive. Though at night I could hear her cry.

Further resilience was needed later the following year, after they returned to London and lost another unborn child, Rory, this time at 22 weeks. Sarah would talk sometimes about her shadow children and one of the chapters addresses how she negotiated this period.

These tragedies marked Sarah deeply but, despite this, she and Kris had one of the best family lives I could imagine. The happiness of their marriage was tangible; their joy at winning at football or the races catching in its exuberance. She adored her parents, her family-in-law, her sister, her brother, their spouses, her nephews and nieces. There were dinners, parties, meals out and trips to the seaside. She cooked huge meals for us, even inviting my family to join her whole family once for Christmas when I had reached the end of my turkey tether. Even though the years of heavy drinking and partying had ceased – Sarah was far more responsible at motherhood than me – she was still always so alive, so much the beating heart of so many gatherings.

November 2017. When it came, the call was abrupt. *They're going to lop off my tit.* This really was a crisis but Sarah made no drama of it. From the off she was as pragmatic as could be. The cancer was aggressive, growing to a tumour of eight centimetres in less than three weeks. Speed was essential and within the month she had started chemotherapy. Kris sent me a photo of her first session – she was fitted with a cold cap, her laptop in front of her as she worked to ensure that she met her latest deadline. She had no intention of letting cancer or its treatment get in the way of her work.

It didn't, though I think it would have felled a lesser person. It would have felled me. I'd have taken to my bed and told my editors there was no way I'd file in time. But even as the chemo spread its poison through her, she kept on going. In every other area, too, she kept on as normal, taking each difficulty in her stride. I remember visiting a few weeks into the treatment to see her with her head shaved – the cold cap hadn't worked and, fed up with handfuls of her hair falling out in the shower, Sarah had gone to the barber round the corner and asked them to get rid of the lot.

This was over three years ago. The treatment plan was brutal but ought to have been effective. Chemotherapy, mastectomy, radiotherapy. She and Kris invited me to dinner in the Cotswolds to celebrate the end of the treatment and we drank rosé at a restaurant in Kingham where their dog Murphy (as beloved as Spurs) was also welcome. When I finish treatment I don't want to do a marathon, she'd said some months before, I want to go on holiday. We went to a villa in Skiathos, an island in the Sporades, and a whole group of friends ate and drank and swam for the happiest of weeks under an Aegean sky.

A period of remission would have been nice.

Sarah had certainly earned it. But it wasn't to be. She had a scan on her return from holiday at the end of the summer, 2018, which carried the worst possible news. The cancer had metastasised, spread to her liver. There wasn't going to be a happy end to this story – recovery was no longer a possibility. The point of treatment now was to extend her life for as long as possible at the highest quality. Barring a miracle, no cure would be possible.

It was Ruby's birthday the next day. It came as no surprise to me to see that it was business as usual at their house, the typical resilience shown by Sarah and Kris still much on display. I was in awe, though. They would have been entirely within their rights to have stopped the clocks, drawn the blinds and refused to come out. But still they persisted. The treatments took their toll but trips out still happened, visits to friends and family. Sarah and I would meet in Chiswick for breakfast most weeks before going to the Waterstones across the road, and I'd inevitably leave with an armful of new books at her recommendation. Despite the rigours of her treatment another holiday was achieved, a dream trip to Jamaica to visit cherished friends.

We talked a lot during that time, about our children, our work. About death. Sarah was never afraid for herself. Maybe because of her upbringing as a Catholic, her faith was a quiet constant in her life, never overwhelming it but deep in her foundations. She was afraid for those she'd leave behind, though.

Then the pandemic hit. The timing couldn't have been more cruel, the fact that so much of what could have happened was so curtailed. No longer was it possible for us to meet for breakfast, or for the happy gatherings of family and friends that had been so important. Sarah's health was also beginning to be badly affected by the treatments, leading to long stays in hospital, where, hardest of all, she was unable to receive any visitors, though Kris spent as much time with her as he possibly could. There were brief interludes of almost normality, too, a family birthday celebration for Oisín in the summer of 2020 a bittersweet joy.

There was so much that Sarah couldn't control. But what she could control was her work. The last three years of Sarah's life were hard beyond imagination in so many respects but her creative output was unstoppable. They say that a tree flowers most extravagantly in the year before its death – Sarah knew her time was short and her work reached its peak during this time. Not just in her list of book recommendations in the *i* that so many of us leaped on as soon as it was published, ready to add even more to our shelves; the book and television reviews that she wrote with such care and expertise; the interviews that she carried out even when she was at her most ill; the blogs she wrote for popular television series – all these were so important, the community of readers she'd built up over the six series of *Line of Duty* a particularly warm and loyal corner of the internet. But it was the way she wrote about her life that I think is her most significant legacy.

Inevitably, this is a book about living with cancer. About dying from it, too. But it's so much more than that. As Sarah described it herself, it's a 'portrait of a life lived well, if carelessly', and how her family coped 'when the good times ran out and bitter reality kicked in'. That bitter reality is confronted head on in the chapter 'Scars', and in Sarah's thoughts on being the first of her friends to die. It's interspersed throughout with humour, though, and with joy. 'In the kingdom of cancer different rules apply', she says at one point, and Sarah was endlessly inventive in finding ways to bring light into the darkness. The chapter on fashion shows exactly this – only Sarah could find the upside in the drastic weight loss brought on by the disease and embrace the opportunity to wear the French fashion she'd craved. Always beautifully turned out in those last years, she had an array of ornate turbans, and photographs from her last birthday in November 2020 show her done up to the nines for a cocktail evening at home with Kris, her children and her beloved goddaughter Sefi.

Even though her own appetite was affected, she found solace in reading about food, too. Her recipe book collection was unsurpassed and she took full advantage of one of the few positive benefits of the pandemic by ordering a wild array of recipe boxes from top restaurants to be delivered to her home and enjoyed by her and her family, captured in loving detail in the chapter 'Food, Confusing Food'. Some of the boxes she ordered didn't arrive until after her death, a celestial benediction to her family by way of pie and spices. She would message from hospital during her interminable stays to ask us to bring food for her; tortilla, Greek salad, *pan bagnat*, deliveries from her dearest friend Sandra a particular favourite.

Like Alexander Hamilton, Sarah wrote like she was running out of time. She achieved so much of her memoir in such a short time. But time did run out. There's so much I wish was different but one of the biggest gaps is that of the chapters left unwritten. I have the original proposal in front of me now, with so many enticing titles there never to be fulfilled. 'Teenage Kicks', which would have touched on the risky behaviour of her teens and early twenties and how Sarah finally grew up. 'Financial Advice from an Unrepentant Gambler', the content of which I can imagine only too well and makes me smile. 'Circle of Friends', which would have been an essay on her friendships, those made and those lost. Most intriguing of all, 'The Secret Lives of Catholic Saints', from her early childhood reading the *Little Book of Martyred Saints*, using the suffering of St Catherine on the wheel to describe the worst moments when Sarah was trapped in a hospital bed.

I think that Sarah would be the first to tell me to stop dwelling on what's missing, though, and be grateful for what she did complete. We are lucky to have it, her words enduring so strongly even now she's gone. At an online memorial a few months after her death, some readings were made from a selection of her articles and from these essays, and it was almost like being in her company again, her voice clear and vibrant still.

We will never know what she had to say in that essay about friends but we all knew that Sarah had a gift for friendship, both in making and in keeping friends. From childhood, through school and university, her work, her time in America, she gathered friends around her and kept them close. In this collection of Sarah's essays, there are also contributions from friends at every stage of her life. We can't fill in what Sarah would have written herself but between us, we hope to give a more complete picture of who Sarah was and why she meant so much to each of us. It's only a few – there could have been so much more.

Tilly Bagshawe writes about meeting Sarah at school, Adrian Berry about their years at university. Alexa Baracaia tells of meeting Sarah in Manchester and Brendan Conellan of her years in New York. Their friendships with Sarah all had different points of genesis but the key similarity is their endurance: all lasted through decades. Most moving of all is the end chapter, written by Kris, Sarah's husband, in which he talks about the good times, the way they found happiness together as a family, even in the saddest of moments.

It's this that is the most important aspect of Sarah's work. Life ends, but it also carries on. 'Love is always about letting go as much as it is about holding tight,' she writes in the chapter 'The Memory Box', which inspired the title to this memoir. Rather than dwelling on everything she had lost through cancer, Sarah focused on what she had. So much in her life was worth celebration. We need to learn from this, to be glad for what we had of her, rather than to dwell on her loss, holding her memory close to us as we move forward into the light that her life has made so much brighter.

It's My Funeral and I'll Cry If I Want To

FROM AN EARLY AGE I WAS OBSESSED BY DEATH. Cursed with a short temper, I was the sort of child who would storm off to my room when angry, where, lying on my bed, I would pass the time imagining my funeral and how devastated my family would be by my premature death.

There was something deeply satisfying about this. Something soothing about imagining such a thoroughly over-the-top scenario, that spoke to my innate sense of the dramatic and tendency towards melodrama.

At nine years old, I spent a lot of time reading

books such as Susan Coolidge's *What Katy Did* but, instead of imagining that having suffered a terrible accident, I would surprise all around me by becoming a 'better' person, thanks to learning to live with the pain, I would picture a terrible car crash or unexpected fall from which I didn't recover but died.

My weeping family would lay me on the bed and peel off my white kid boots and smart cream coat, removing my blood-stained fur muff from my hand – for some reason, my nine-year-old self envisaged a world in which I died dressed like the period dolls my father bought back from trips to America – and they wouldn't stop crying until the moment they laid me in my cold, dark grave. And perhaps not even then.

Every year, they would visit my sad little grave, bringing flowers and discussing how much they missed me and how much they wished they'd been more understanding when I was alive.

As for me, I would haunt the house like a sad Victorian ghost child, my faint footsteps echoing through the hallways of our Edinburgh home, causing people to look up and say 'Was that possibly . . . ? No, it can't be', before returning to their meal with a vague sense of unease (I had also been reading a lot of ghost stories at this time in addition to my much-thumbed-through copy of Usborne's *The World of the Unknown: Ghosts*).

Later that year, I watched the 1949 version of *Little Women* starring June Allyson as Jo March, Janet Leigh as Meg, Margaret O'Brien as Beth and Elizabeth Taylor as Amy. When I had read Louisa May Alcott's book I had pictured myself as Jo – doesn't every book-loving child? – but watching the film, I realised that it wasn't Jo I most wanted to be but quiet, unassuming Beth who gets the big death scene, the hushed house, the grieving family.

Personality-wise we might have nothing in common but I thrilled to the idea of being the person whose death changes everything, forcing her sisters to make decisions they might otherwise not have made. These days, I realise that the meek and delicate Beth would never have thought about or planned her death, and my love for melodrama and flair for the dramatic, my desire to be noticed and mourned by all makes me Amy instead. I've come to terms with it.

~

As I grew older, so my obsession with death grew more intense. When I was aged ten, my parents sent me to boarding school on the Sussex coast, more because my dad thought it was the right thing to do rather than out of any strong belief in the importance of the system. It was an error which he has said he regrets.

Chafing against the rules around bedtime, the sharing of dorms and, worst of all, the prohibition regarding what TV could be watched (the horror of not being allowed to watch my favourite series, the Second World War prisoner of war drama *Tenko*), I returned home and told my dad I hated boarding school and felt as though I was being punished. Without pause he hugged me, said, 'Well then, you can leave,' and that was that. I'd lasted a term.

There were some good things to come out of those dark and lonely weeks on the cold, wet coast, however – chiefly the fact that I discovered the novels of Daphne Du Maurier.

Sitting on the window ledge of my dormitory at weekends when the other girls had gone home – with my family living in Scotland, I was often stuck there with the small group of ex-pats, all of us eagerly grasping at the occasional invite to other girls' houses – I devoured *Rebecca*, *My Cousin Rachel*, *The Parasites* and *The King's General*.

My funeral fantasies took a turn for the gothic. Now, instead of simpering choirs of angels and white coffins, I imagined black plumed horses, mourners in jet necklaces, veils and rosary beads, cameos of the dead pinned to black shirts for remembrance. It would rain on the day of the funeral and mourners would fight to keep their umbrellas open in the wind as they lowered my black coffin into the ground. Perhaps, like the Victorians, some of my friends would preserve a piece of my hair in an amber locket and think of me when they were having fun.

A couple of years later, I started a new secondary school in Edinburgh and began the standard teenage experimentation: trying new styles, applying copious amounts of black eyeliner, taking up smoking and, best of all, gathering with friends to pass drink around in the nearby cemetery after school. The lack of mobile phones allowed us to excuse our late return with the barely believable but brazenly delivered excuse that the 41 bus was late, once again.

I discovered Charles Dickens's *Bleak House* and imagined myself as Lady Dedlock 'bored to death' and 'quite out of temper' in her rain-sodden Lincolnshire home. Reading of Krook's spectacularly over-the-top death in the same book, I passed hours wondering if it was really possible to die of spontaneous combustion? How would people react if all they found was a pile of ashes where you once sat? Would they believe that you had gone or think you'd simply run away?

No sooner had I come to terms with the sheer unlikeliness of ending life in this way than a new, more fascinating form of death presented itself thanks to F. Scott Fitzgerald.

Reading about the American novelist's tuberculosis, I pictured a world in which I was sent to Switzerland for a cure, pushed out daily from the ward to catch the healthy rays of the Swiss sun, only for the disease to persist. Sent back home, I would subsequently languish on a chaise longue, feeling faint and pressing my bloodstained handkerchief to my mouth as I received a stream of distraught visitors and slowly wasted away.

This, it seemed, was finally the ideal death: protracted, fraught with the possibility of recovery and then relapse, guaranteed to arouse sympathy, not of my making. Even better, it was not an entirely impossible end. I had a positive Mantoux test, which meant that I had come into some contact with TB and couldn't have the BCG jab given as standard to all Scottish secondary school pupils. My furious mother, an infection control doctor, was convinced I had scratched the test scab to make it rise up, only to be told by my father that he had had contact with TB when younger and this was probably the reason for my positive test.

Vindicated, I headed to the hospital, preparing my dying swan act as I went. Unfortunately, reality is rarely as exciting as the imagination and six months of weekly lung scans swiftly put paid to any notion of the disease as romantic. Not only did I not have TB but I realised I really didn't want it.

∾

It would be nice to say that the whole experience cured me of my death fantasies but it wasn't really true. Instead, I would spend hours sitting on the window ledge of my room dangling my legs over while smoking and wondering what would happen if I allowed myself to let go and fall.

Once, I even went as far as to loop the curtain cord round my neck while my parents relaxed outside in the garden on one of those all-too-rare sunlit Edinburgh days. My monstrous (and monstrously self-obsessed) hope was that they would look up and, thinking I was trying to kill myself, dash up the stairs. Looking back, I'm really not sure what I was hoping to achieve, given the more likely outcome was that they'd shout at me and, in shock, I'd slip and actually kill myself, as opposed to pretending to.

I read 'Resumé', Dorothy Parker's infamous poem on different methods of suicide and spent a considerable amount of time pondering which would be the best way to die: razor, rope, pills, or should I simply take heed of the dry conclusion that you 'might as well live'?

Worst of all, I wrote screeds of bad teenage poetry about death, including the memorably awful: 'Here marks the spot where she lay/Once death came for her and bore her away/Time's winged chariot passing by/She surrendered life without a cry.' That I can still remember the opening over 30 years later is testament to how dreadful a poem it was. Inexplicably, the school put it up on the wall as an example of good work.

It was around this time too that I became obsessed by the Scottish border ballad 'The Daemon Lover', a.k.a. 'James Herries', with its haunting final verse: 'O what a black, dark hill is yon/That looks so dark to me?/O it is the hill of hell, he said/ Where you and I shall be.'

I would listen to Johnny Cash's version of 'Long Black Veil' and other country murder ballads on repeat and replay the Scottish folk song 'Helen of Kirkconnel' – 'Oh, curs'd the heart that thought the thought/And curs'd the hand that fired the shot/When in my arms my Helen dropped/And died for sake o' me' – with the same fervour that, as an older teen, I played Sinéad O'Connor's devastating cover of 'I Am Stretched on Your Grave'.

I read too of Koschei the Deathless, the Slavic demon buying immortality with young women; of Mesopotamian goddess Ishtar descending into the underworld to save her lost love and Egyptian goddess Isis doing the same to find her missing husband Osiris.

In my late teens, my family moved back to London and I spent a considerable amount of time tramping through various London cemeteries from Kensal Rise to Highgate. I read Anne Billson's witty vampire novel *Suckers*, where a pretentious

young photographer depicts his girlfriends looking mournful in those very venues and was thrilled
by James Hogg's *The Private Memoirs and Con-
fessions of a Justified Sinner* with its souls saved
and damned.

None of this, however, was real. Yes, there were
times when I took a razor and made marks on my
skin but I resorted to that more as a release from
pent-up teenage emotions. The cuts were shallow and my intentions less suicidal than hormone
driven – my hormones raged like an unstoppable
bushfire for most of my teens, causing me to want
to scream, shout, slam doors and generally flounce.
Using the razor stopped those tensions from roil-
ing inside me for a while but I soon realised that
I wasn't serious, not a dedicated cutter like the
handful of anxiety-driven, genuinely unwell girls
at various schools I attended, whose cuts marked
their entire bodies, deep and desperate cries for
help. Ashamed by the notion that I was playing at
something so serious, I stopped. Similarly, I might
have thought a lot about Parker's methods for suicide, read about Edgar Allen Poe's Annabel Lee

languishing 'in her tomb by the sounding sea' or wondered what it would be like to have my very own marble mausoleum like the ones in Highgate, but I never actually considered killing myself. I enjoyed life far too much and had no real interest in dying. It was death itself, the process, the funeral, the possibility of an afterlife, the way in which those left behind moved on, or didn't, that fascinated me.

In any story there is always one friend who dies earlier than expected, whose death is shocking, who is destined to be referenced by the rest as age descends upon them. Who haunts their conversations when they think back to good times gone and start to imagine what that person would have been like in middle or old age. Throughout my twenties I wondered who that person might be. Which of us was doomed to be the one struck by tragedy? Who would go first? One of my wild friends who drank heavily and partied long into the night fuelled by drugs and music? Or one of the quieter ones, taken by accident, walking out one day and for some terrible reason never coming home? The surprising answer was none of them.

People I knew did die, in motorcycle crashes and of sudden unexplained brain haemorrhages, but they were friends of friends rather than people I knew well. My inner circle, the people I loved, lived and laughed through our twenties and thirties, untouched by tragedy, lucky souls.

I married and spent rather more time than was healthy wondering what would happen if my husband, Kris, suddenly dropped dead and how devastated I would be. I planned an alternative life in which my children and I were forced to live a very different way, lacking the person who held us all together, made us laugh, kept everything going even when we drove him insane.

I imagined the deaths of my children, my parents, siblings and various friends. I experienced the true horror of death when I grieved two stillborn children, a roaring emptiness clawing at my insides, my wild emotions constantly threatening to burst through my skin. Yet still I wondered, who is it who will die (relatively) young? Which of us will go first?

As the ancient gods would tell you, be careful what you're thinking. Mythology and folklore are littered with the stories of those who believed they could cheat death or make bargains for their souls. They never end well.

Thus, at the age of 45, when I had long moved on from dreams of death, when I was happily married with two small children, when I still remembered my dead babies but without the raw anger that had once threatened to overwhelm, death, the dancer I had tempted and taunted all my life, finally heeded my unconscious invitation and knocked at my door.

At first, the cancer diagnosis seemed straightforward. Yes, the lump in my breast was large and yes, it had spread to couple of lymph nodes. But it's part of human nature to be hopeful and everyone I talked to after that first diagnosis was confident that all would be well.

Plenty of other women I knew had found lumps. They had undergone often gruelling treatment but they had survived. Months later now, their hair was growing back, the cancer was gone, they had begun to rebuild their lives.

OK, so my particular cancer was triple negative, arguably the most difficult to treat, and the tumour did appear to be particularly aggressive but that was no reason to despair. Everyone I talked to at the busy west London hospital where I was treated was confident. The next few months would be hard but we would get through them and move on.

It didn't quite work out like that. Initially the signs were good. The aggressive chemotherapy worked. The tumour shrunk away to nothing. The mastectomy operation and breast reconstruction went well. They removed 27 lymph nodes from my left arm and none had cancer in them. Everyone was delighted with what looked like the best possible result – I just needed to wait for my breast to heal before having radiation to target the one lymph node that couldn't be removed due to its location near an artery on the other side of my breast.

It's here that everything started to go wrong. I didn't realise at first. The breast healed. The radiotherapy was completed. I had a lovely two-week holiday with friends at a villa on the Greek island of Skiathos and returned feeling refreshed, healthy – my hair was growing back thick and, to my surprise, curly; my eyebrows and eyelashes had returned. I felt ready for the rest of my life.

Then a weekly check-up found that the tumour markers were going back up. A PET scan confirmed the worst: it had been a tiny possibility but, at some point, probably between the breast healing and the start of radiotherapy, a cancerous cell had merrily travelled down my bloodstream to my liver where it began to multiply. Adding to the problem, it chose to do this not by forming one big tumour but instead by spreading in tiny bits all over the liver, rather like freckles across a face.

I had gone from being cancer free to having stage IV or metastatic cancer. In other words: incurable. For what remained of my life, I would be living with a chronic disease. Thirty-one people die every day from metastatic cancer – a horrifying statistic that has powered the important MetUp campaign, which draws attention to how little provision and thought is given to those living with metastatic cancer with the stark slogan: Dying for a Cure.

For we really are. The odds are particularly terrible for triple negative metastatic patients. On average, we die less than a year after our diagnosis. No wonder my oncologist told me to enjoy life as much as I could and take as many holidays as possible (a lesson I took to heart, heading off on family trips to Rome, Jamaica and, thanks to the kindness of friends and the organisation of one of my sister's best friends in particular, a wonderful trip to New York that was filled with catch-ups with old friends and memorable new experiences).

Before all that, however, I sat in her room as my world caved in and tried to absorb the news. It was at that moment I realised I had the answer to my long-pondered question: the person who was going to die first from my friendship group was me.

e⁓

Incredibly, I made it past that first tough year. It is now three years since I received the metastatic cancer diagnosis and during that time, I have had countless treatments from chemotherapies to Sirtex radiation of the liver. I have developed ascites, necessitating the fitting of a PleurX drain and giving poor Kris yet another task in the shape of draining the liquid out of my stomach every day.

I have contracted sepsis, visited A&E, been emergency admitted semi-conscious and unaware of my surrounding and come close to dying when a varicose vein almost burst, leading to an endoscopy and the fitting of preventative bands on said vein. I have struggled with my bowels, spent nights feeling unbelievably sick and realised that morphine makes me perky rather than knocks me out. Throughout it all I have lived.

In doing so, I have come to realise how very lucky I am to have an incredible support system and, most of all, an unflappable husband who is still able to laugh about our situation and two sanguine children who largely take what is happening in their increasingly competent stride.

I plan my funeral, too. All those years dreaming about death weren't entirely wasted, it turns out, and one benefit of knowing that you have finite time on earth and that you will probably have some warning of when you will die is being able to work out exactly how you want to say goodbye.

I want a big party in my house with everyone dressed up and the music playing long into the night. I will wear a fancy turban, a black Sicilian widow's dress and big boots. And if I have to hop around drinking liquid morphine from a hip flask like the playwright Dennis Potter in his final interview with Melvyn Bragg in 1994 then I will. The next morning, early, I want to drive with Kris, the children and the dog to Brighton where I will sit on the stony beach and eat fish and chips while drinking a glass of champagne and staring out at the turbulent sea I have always adored.

I want a proper Irish wake with my body laid out, plates of sandwiches and cigarettes and people coming to share a toast and memories. I want at least one person to accidentally put their whiskey tumbler on the coffin and leave an indelible stain. Having never quite grown out of my youthful wallowing, I still want those black-plumed horses and that old-fashioned Victorian funeral display. At the funeral itself, I want Patrick Kavanagh's 'On Raglan Road' and the old Irish classic 'Carrickfergus' to be sung, and some of my favourite poems read, including Louis MacNeice's 'The Sunlight on the Garden', Dylan Thomas's 'And Death Shall Have No Dominion', John Betjeman's 'Sun and Fun' and W. B. Yeats's 'The Circus Animals' Desertion'. The service will end with Sandy Denny's 'Who Knows Where the Time Goes' because I have always liked to cry so why not make everyone else join me?

Because I am an unashamed drama queen, I wish to record a goodbye message to be played at the reception, which should be filled with laughter and booze and good food and high spirits. And yes, I have made a playlist, filled with loud songs and quiet, with country and folk and hip hop and pop, with reggae and rap and indie and rock. It's a soundtrack to get people dancing and singing, to sing along to and to remember me by.

I want people to remember the good times and the terrible, the mad and sad moments, and those where we gasped for laughter and wept until we thought we'd never stop. Because to misquote Lesley Gore's 1963 classic: 'It's my funeral and I'll cry if I want to. You would cry too, if it happened to you.'

Sarah's Teenage Years
by Tilly Bagshawe

I FIRST MET SARAH IN SEPTEMBER 1989. We were both 16 and starting sixth form at Woldingham School, a deeply traditional, conservative, middle-class, all-girl, Catholic boarding school in leafy suburban Surrey. I had already spent the past two years there, doing my GCSEs. Sarah was new. She'd been expelled from at least one school by that point I believe – Fettes College in Edinburgh and perhaps one other esteemed private establishment, paid for at great expense by her devoted and (by this point, presumably) faintly despairing parents. In any event, she arrived at Woldingham that

September, a wild, unbroken Irish mare in a school full of blonde, identikit dressage ponies. Sarah did not, on any level whatsoever, fit in. I really can't stress that enough.

We became friends immediately.

After Sarah's death, when I read all the many tributes to her from fans of her writing around the world, I was amused to discover that within the *Game of Thrones* community, she had been known as 'Lady Sarah'. Not amused because she was anything less than a lady, in the sense of being noble and brilliant and really just marvellous in every way – she was all of those things. But because the Sarah I knew, and certainly the teenage Sarah, was not remotely lady*like*. And I think the feminist in her – the wild, ferocious, uncompromising feminist – would have baulked violently at the whole idea of being termed a 'lady'. That was not something Sarah aspired to.

Woldingham girls were 'ladies'. They, at least the popular ones among them, had blonde hair that they flicked coquettishly, went out with rugby-playing public schoolboys called Sebastian or

Piers or Torquil, longed to be photographed for the society pages of *Tatler* and spent inordinate amounts of time shaving their legs, plucking their eyebrows and learning about the opposite sex from the problem pages of *Cosmo*. The posters on their walls were of Jason Donovan or Patrick Swayze in *Dirty Dancing* and the rebels among them hid miniatures of Malibu under their pillows and occasionally indulged in a puff or two on a Silk Cut Light.

I say 'them' but, truth be told, I was one of them in many ways. Not wholly. But in the grand Venn diagram of the teenage experience, our lives certainly intersected.

Sarah's life did not. She had about as much in common with the rest of our classmates as Priti Patel has with Jeremy Corbyn, or Katie Price with Albert Einstein. Sarah smoked Marlboro Reds – packets and packets of them. She drank whiskey, claret or snakebite and black. She loathed women's magazines and their advice columns that suggested girls pretend to be unable to carry their suitcases so that boys would do it for them (and presumably be charmed by their feminine vulnerability). Everything Sarah knew about the opposite sex she learned by shagging them. Nor could she be remotely arsed to shave her legs first. Also by beating them in debates, and at cards, and in exams, and at everything, really.

Sarah was quite simply a force of nature, like no one any of us had ever met. Or at least, not outside of the pages of the Jilly Cooper novels that she and I both devoured like acolytes of some brilliant, wildly aspirational cult. As a teenager, Sarah *was* Caitlin O'Hara from Cooper's *Rivals*. Charming, rebellious, clever, kind, funny, Irish and sexy, albeit in her own, rather militant way. I remember her in those early years of our friendship with a curtain of dark hair flopping over her eyes and a fag permanently clamped between her lips. She wore a uniform of ripped black tights, a miniscule miniskirt and scuffed Doc Marten boots, and spent most of her time reading, drinking, quoting Yeats, cackling with profoundly unladylike laughter and generally being the life and soul of the party while confidently spouting absolute nonsense much of the time, as teenagers are wont to do. She was so cool, so clever and so *tough*, at least on the outside. To this day, I have friends from Woldingham who remember Sarah as the 'brilliant girl with the rhinoceros hide', the 'witty outsider' who 'didn't give a shit'.

But, of course, she did give a shit. Beneath that 'rhinoceros hide' Sarah was sensitive and, yes, even vulnerable; and I think she suffered quite deeply from the casual spite and bitchiness that she encountered from certain groups of girls at school. The popular cliques were threatened and offended by Sarah's uncompromising, almost masculine manner. By her bluntness, her profound lack of interest in fashion or make-up, her unapologetic intellectualism and her totally liberated sexuality. She *was* an outsider, by choice but perhaps also by necessity, by nature, and she understood what being an outsider meant and how painful and lonely it could be.

The empathy and kindness that her legions of readers and fans praised in her writing as an adult, and that everybody who knew her well rightly

identified as a central pillar of her character –
much of that, I believe, was forged in her teenage
years. Boarding school, with its pointless rules and
stifling traditions, felt ludicrous to Sarah. Because
it *was* ludicrous. As two 16-year-old girls who
knew everything, she and I agreed about that.

Much has been written, and rightly so, about
Sarah's courage. Not just through her cancer and
in facing the prospect of her own death, but in
everything she did, always. 'Brave' is certainly a
word that I strongly associate with her. 'Loyal'
would be another one. 'Kind' a third. But if I had
to pick just *one* adjective to sum up my friend,
I think it would have to be 'funny'. I don't think
I have ever in my life laughed harder or more
often than I have with Sarah. And that all started
in our teens.

I remember one exeat weekend at school; we
had lied as usual to the nuns about going to stay
with somebody's maiden aunt or grandmother in
Bognor Regis (this was in the halcyon days before
mobile phones or internet so nobody could check
anything, and horrible, deceitful teenagers like

Sarah and me were taken at our word) and then snuck off to London together in search of adventure. We got as far as the Admiral Codrington pub in South Kensington, with no money, no plan and, potentially problematically, no place to stay for the night.

By around ten, I was starting to get a bit nervous. Last orders were approaching and we still had nowhere to sleep, having failed to bump into anyone we knew.

'Leave it to me,' said Sarah confidently. 'This always works.'

She proceeded to slump down across the bar, flinging her arms out wide, and start gasping violently and very dramatically for breath, wheezing with the most godawful death rattle.

Inevitably the two young men sitting nearest to us rushed over.

'Are you alright?' they asked, panicked. 'What is it? What's the matter?'

At which point Sarah raised her head, fixed them with a gimlet stare, and drawled, deadpan: 'I'm dying.'

'Dying?'

'Yes,' Sarah gasped. 'Of thirst.'

It could have gone either way. But luckily for us, the boys found it hilarious, bought us both drinks and ended up putting us up for the night – quite chastely, I might add – on their fold-out sofa in Fulham. We were idiots of course. Anything could have happened. But what *did* in fact happen was that Sarah's wit and charm and brass balls saved our bacon.

This sort of living on the edge was new and thrilling for me but it was evidently *de rigueur* for Sarah, who approached these types of situations with breathtaking insouciance. I think this was a quality she inherited from her father, Sean, with whom she had an incredibly close bond as a teenager. I was also a daddy's girl but my father was very much on a pedestal, whereas Sarah's was more of a partner in crime, at least in her eyes. I remember her dad taking us both to a fancy dinner at the Dorchester on Park Lane for Sarah's eighteenth birthday and the two of them just coming alive in one another's company, talking books and history and Irish politics and religion and God knows what else. The only other person who I ever saw her that happy with was another Irishman, more than a decade later, who thankfully she ended up marrying, because they were perfect for each other.

I think Sarah was drawn to me initially for the same reasons I was drawn to her. We were both clever and ambitious, both feminists and both rebellious, with a pronounced naughty streak. When I got pregnant at 17 and decided to keep the baby, Sarah was a thousand per cent supportive. When I asked her to be my daughter Sefi's godmother, she accepted, but with the matter-of-fact disclaimer that, 'I'll be shit when she's a baby. I find babies really boring. But when she's a fucked-up teenager with drug problems and a massively unsuitable boyfriend, I'll be amazing.' And by God, she was.

She had two young children of her own by that point and had tragically also lost two others, a daughter and a son, to late miscarriage and stillbirth. The bravery with which she bore those twin griefs, and the openness and honesty with which she spoke about them, said so much about the person that Sarah was. But her capacity for love and emotional generosity were limitless, and she welcomed Sefi into her life without hesitation.

Throughout my daughter's troubled and often chaotic young adulthood, Sarah was the ultimate friend – kind, available and honest but never judgmental, patient to a degree I never would have believed her capable of when we were younger, and often wasn't capable of myself. It's no exaggeration to say that she became a second mother to Sefi through these years. Sef loved her fiercely in return and had the huge privilege of being with Sarah when she died, at home as she had wanted to, holding her hand alongside Sarah's husband Kris.

By that point, physically, Sarah had become a shadow of the girl I knew. But her wit and intellect were as razor sharp as ever. The last time I saw her in person was just after Christmas 2020, when we went for a walk in a local field with our respective kids and Sarah's psychotic, appallingly trained but ridiculously endearing dog, Murphy. She was so frail that Kris had to hold her up at times while she ranted about Boris's pandemic incompetence and we debated Joe 'Everybody's Third Choice since 1974!' Biden. I told her her bald head made her look like Gollum. She told me to fuck off. It was a nice afternoon but Sarah was in pain and exhausted by the time we said goodbye. I knew it was unlikely I would see her again. Or at least, not until she'd blagged her way past St Peter at the Pearly Gates. And assuming that she had enough blarney to get me in as well.

Sarah never changed fundamentally from the girl she was when I met her at 16. Her life changed, of course. And she blossomed, and matured, and became a (wonderful) mother, and writer, and all of those things. But she never altered the way that *she* was to fit in with the world or to meet the expectations of others. Not at Woldingham. Not afterwards. Not ever.

I don't believe many people can say that.

What Trashy Novels Taught Me About Life

IT WAS THE COVERS THAT FIRST DREW ME IN. Four children staring out in fear, seemingly trapped behind a window, someone somewhere clearly wishing them harm; a girl with long hair in a Victorian nightdress menaced by a giant red-and-green plant.

I turned the novels over in my hands in the Edinburgh department store. What were these books? At 12 I'd never seen anything like them. Checking that my parents and siblings were still shopping elsewhere, I settled down on the floor and cracked open the spines. Later I would beg my mum to let me buy them. Bemused, she agreed.

Virginia Andrews's *Flowers in the Attic* is the cocaine of trashy novels – easily consumed, delivering rollercoaster highs and lows, leaving a slightly bitter aftertaste. The main message appears to be: 'Don't worry if your previously lovely mother suddenly reveals herself to be a deranged psychopath who locks you and your siblings in the attic before deciding to poison you all with sugared doughnuts. As long as you can have sex with your hot twin brother everything will turn out for the best in the end.'

Incredibly, Andrews's *My Sweet Audrina*, possibly the only novel in the world to feature a vengeful former ice-skating champion who is now a double leg amputee confined to a little red trolley, is even more ludicrously plotted. It features multiple memories, girls with eyes like 'prisms', hints of terrible things that happened in the woods near the heroine's house and arguably the finest description of how not to handle childhood trauma ever committed to page.

'Don't lie to your children' is a pretty good lesson but it was still clear, even to my 12-year-old self, that Andrews was not the ideal author to learn about life from. What she was, however, was a gateway to another world.

It's easy to mock so-called 'trashy' novels. People do it all the time. They're dismissed as bonkbusters and shagathons. Laughed at for their over-the-top prose. Characterised as being about nothing more than sex and shopping. To their many detractors, they are sugary book bonbons, the gilded covers with their (often one-word) titles raised up on the front – *Lace*, *Rivals*, *Scandal*, *Lucky* – further signs that these books lack purpose. They are 'women's fiction', frivolous works, not the sort of thing a serious reader should bother with.

Those critics are wrong. There is much to learn within the pages of the so-called bonkbuster – and, no, not all of it is about sex. These are books filled with wit and hard-won wisdom. They are the books that taught me about female friendship and ambition. Careers are important in these stories, as is love – but not always in the sense of 'and then she got married and lived happily ever after'. They are books about taking risks and putting yourself out there, stuffed full of heroines who have never heard of impostor syndrome but who instead get up, put their game face on, stride out and remake the world in their image day after day after day.

Yes, they are also full of fashion tips and make-up recommendations – but fashion is not a frivolous business and the way in which women apply make-up or their clothes choices can be filled with meaning and intent. It is true it's a trope of the genre to name-drop designers and that too many of the best-known authors, from Jilly Cooper to Judith Krantz, were uncomfortably obsessed with weight and the notion of the ugly-duckling-to-beautiful-swan transformation.

Yet for all those 'But Miss Jones, you are beautiful' moments, there is something truly awe-inspiring about the 1980s heroine in full fight. Reading these stories in my early teens, I knew I would never grow up to be Jackie Collins's tempestuous Lucky Santangelo, mafia boss's daughter and killer operative in her own right. I probably wouldn't create my own shopping empire from nothing, like the redoubtable Emma Harte in Barbara Taylor

Bradford's *A Woman of Substance*. Nor even negotiate my move to British TV while showing off my 'rapacious' body to good effect in a bright yellow sheath dress, like the fierce and furious television producer Cameron Cook in Cooper's *Rivals*. When I first read the wonderful *Rivals* I adored schoolgirl Caitlin O'Hara, who was the same age as me, but have subsequently come to realise that these days, rather tragically, I most identify with her slatternly mother, Maud, who neglects everything – children, husband, long-lost career, housework – in favour of rereading her favourite novels, eating, drinking and occasionally sloping off for bouts of hot sex.

I might never do anything half as exciting as the torrid events that unfurled in front of my eager eyes as I read long into the night but I can still say with confidence that, for all their supposed lack of seriousness, all that apparent frivolity or even sentimentality, everything I ever learned about life I learned from 'trashy' novels.

After the Andrews epiphany, I began to realise that there must be more books like this out there. The mid-to-late 1980s was a time before young adult fiction; a world of unregulated reading where you jumped from the safety of the children's fiction cocoon, where even the darkest and most nightmarish of tales still felt strangely warming, to the unregulated Wild West of adult fiction where anything could – and it swiftly transpired did – happen.

It was my particular good fortune to be a voracious reader in a family of people who like books but are not entirely obsessed by them. This meant I could cajole everyone into giving me their library cards, which in turn meant I could check out around 12–15 books a week depending on how generous they were feeling. I was lucky, too, that the librarians at Newington Library were the sort of people to turn a blind eye to which books you were checking out, never once telling me that something was unsuitable or 'too old' for me to read.

For a few happy months I ploughed my way through the three great 'J's of bonkbuster fiction – Jackie Collins, Jilly Cooper and Judith Krantz – before supplementing them with a fourth – the highly addictive June Flaum Singer, whose stories of American debutantes gone bad thrilled me to the bone. I discovered Barbara Taylor Bradford (never BTB, not even to fans), Rona Jaffe, Rex Reed, Dominick Dunne, Lisa Alther, Jacqueline Susann and Elizabeth Adler. Then came unsuccessful flings with Sidney Sheldon and Harold Robbins, whose more muscular prose never won my heart.

Then I discovered *Lace*. These days, if you mention Shirley Conran's almost 650-page opus to people they'll come back with one of two things: the moment in the mini-series when Phoebe Cates's Lili hisses: 'Which one of you bitches is my mother?' or the infamous goldfish scene, a.k.a. the moment that thousands of teenage girls in the 1980s debated unto death – 'Yeah, but honestly, how do you think it would feel?'

Yet Conran's book was always more interesting and more serious in intent than those isolated moments, however iconic, suggest. At its heart, *Lace* is a novel about two things: female friendship and feminism. It's a book in which men barely play a role – and where they are centre stage it's often in an uncomfortably exoticised and eroticised way. It's not a novel about marriage or children or finding 'the one', but rather a tale of the importance of having female friends, finding self-worth and being taken seriously in a world that operates in favour of men.

Its four heroines – Judy, Pagan, Maxine and Kate – meet in the confines of a Swiss finishing school after the Second World War. Only one – Judy, who works as a waitress at the local hotel rather than attending the school – is not privileged and yet, as Conran carefully shows, that privilege is not enough to protect them from the world they enter, particularly if they want to work rather than settle down.

Conran goes on to dedicate much of the book to tracking those attempts at forging a career, even as the story's secret – which of the four women got pregnant during their time in Switzerland and what has happened to the subsequent baby – bubbles underneath.

The key line in *Lace*, however, is not that memorable insult from Lili but rather the four girls' schoolroom motto – that they would stick together through 'thick and thin' or, rather, as the French Maxine, perhaps more correctly, has it 'sick and sin'. It is no spoiler to say that is exactly what they do.

Conran had no interest in the alpha bitch grinding rivals under her 10-inch heels. Her book might well be 600-plus pages of sex, success and sensual awakenings, but it is also an honest and heartfelt celebration of the importance of female friends. *Lace* was a revelation in that it showed me there were lessons to be learned from within those gold embossed covers and I took that central one to heart, acknowledging that, yes, there will always be times when your closest friends drive you insane, but there's a reason they are your friends and that's generally because they're with you, making you laugh during both good times and bad.

All these books, even the worst of them, showed me something about life. They were fun reads and often frivolous ones, but inside each there was a kernel of wisdom that you could grab and hold tight to while you were navigating those difficult teenage years. Yes, that was true even of *Flowers in the Attic*. Though given that its message is no matter how terrible your mother turns out to be, don't sleep with your twin brother, I'm not sure how universal a tip that might be.

SEX, LOVE AND FRIENDSHIP: THE RULES OF LIFE ACCORDING TO TRASHY NOVELS

1. Never trust a man with no sense of humour. We might think of the heroes of Jilly Cooper's Rutshire Chronicles as being thrusting, horsey types forever ravaging women in bushes – and to be fair, they often are. But they also know their way around a good quip and most of them are more interested in laughing a woman into bed than presumptuously sweeping her there (you know you've landed a bounder in Jillyshire if they lack a GSOH and are cruel to or, almost worst, indifferent about animals).

2. Live life to the fullest. Jackie Collins showed me you can only get from life what you put in. Her heroines, from mob queen Lucky Santangelo to pop star Venus Maria, barrel through life at maximum speed, grabbing what they can get with both hands and getting away with it because of verve, flair and a sense that this full-throttle existence is the only way to be truly happy.

3. Fashion matters. Reading *The Thorn Birds*, Colleen McCullough's epic tale of love in the Australian outback, what lingered longest was not the doomed central love affair but rather the ashes-of-roses dress that Meggie wears – it was the first time I realised fashion could fuel fantasy. It can send a message, too – *Lace* perfectly captures an era of great change, in part by showing how women threw off the constraints of the past to embrace the youthful fashions of Mary Quant and Biba.

4. Never be afraid of your ambition. It doesn't matter how small your start in life – you could be an overworked teenage servant at a grand house like Emma Harte in Barbara Taylor Bradford's *A Woman of Substance* – it's what you make of it that counts. By the end of the book, Emma heads up a retail empire and her biggest headache is working out which of her many children or grandchildren to leave it all to. Retail is actually a major theme of 1980s sagas and never more so than in Judith Krantz's *Scruples*, which introduced me to one of my favourite bonkbuster tropes: there's nothing so bad in life that it can't be solved by opening your own shop. Don't worry if you're not sure about how or whether it will survive past the simple act of opening, it is enough to have put the razzle-dazzle back in your life. Anyway, once you open it, they will come.

5. It's OK to be unlikable. Two later authors, Penny Vincenzi and Sally Beauman, introduced me to the notion that a heroine can slip up, make mistakes and even openly choose to do the wrong thing. In *Dark Angel*, Beauman's anti-heroine Constance is shown more as a force of nature than a relatable protagonist. First referenced almost as a bad fairy at a disastrous christening, she is later shown to be damaged, deceitful and quite possibly deluded, but she is also one of the most vibrant, compelling characters ever committed to page. Reading about her made me realise that not everything exists in black and white, that most of us inhabit the grey worlds in between. Similarly, Vincenzi's Celia in *No Angel* is autocratic, demanding and selfish, but she also has a clear purpose – the preservation of her beloved publishing house – which often (although not always) justifies even her worst actions. Vincenzi wasn't interested in creating a heroine you simply rooted for. Instead, she gives us something much more complex: a woman you don't always like but who feels believable.

6. It's also OK to fail. Long before the current plethora of podcasts and books about the art of failing there was Ginny Babcock. The heroine of *Kinflicks*, Lisa Alther's bawdy romp of a book, is a bad daughter, failed cheerleader, sexually confused scion of 1960s America and a woman who spends her life trying on a series of different personas, permanently dissatisfied because none of them quite seems to fit. Ginny's life is one long stream of failure – in that sense, *Kinflicks* is as much the female answer to John Kennedy Toole's *A Confederacy of Dunces* as it is a true bonkbuster – punctuated by scenes of eye-popping sex, some good but most often bad. As a 15-year-old, I snorted my way through it, eagerly turning its pages to see what misfortune would befall Ginny next. As an adult, I realise that Alther's strength lies in the way she allows her heroine to fail without judgement. Like every good bonkbuster heroine, Ginny picks herself up after each disaster and carries on.

7. And to enjoy sex... Rona Jaffe's *Class Reunion* showed me a woman doesn't have to be afraid of her sexual appetite. Her gorgeous, free-spirited heroine Annabel Jones is initially punished for enjoying her sexual encounters at university but Jaffe makes very clear that this is a problem with 1950s American morality, not with Annabel herself. Of all her four heroines it is Annabel who eventually creates the most contented life. The implication is that it is because Annabel is comfortable in her body and knows who she is and what she likes that she lives a happy and fulfilled life. Elsewhere, Rita Mae Brown's raucous *Rubyfruit Jungle* showed me love and sex didn't just have to be between a woman and a man, while Lesley Lokko's smart and addictive *Sundowners* taught me you should never be afraid to express your opinions, even if it means that the boy you fancy might see you in a different, less flattering, light.

St Andrews
by Adrian Berry

1991

SARAH HITS ST ANDREWS UNIVERSITY IN 1991. With irresistible force, the immovable object is struck. She has been cannon-shot from a Catholic boarding school into the citadel of Scotland's Protestant reformation. The counter-reformation is about to begin.

St Andrews is golf courses, a university, a harbour with a few fishing boats, and home to the poor souls of Fife who depend on one or other of them. The university is so old it has four history departments (ancient, medieval, modern and Scottish) but no present. There is no Thatcherite consumer revolution reaching here. And the prospect of a Scottish Parliament is the stuff of patriotic fantasy. To enter the Criterion Bar on South Street is to enter a world that could be any time from the 1950s onwards. To sit in the Old Union Diner, the student café near the arts faculty, amid the cigarette smoke and talk of essays undone, is to be held fast in a world preserved in illusory amber.

On the dark ceiling beams of the diner are embossed the names of the university's rectors. From J. S. Mill through to Rudyard Kipling and Field Marshal Haig, and onwards to the mundane, post-war world. It's the story of 'great men' and it's over. But no one has told them. Sitting beneath them on a hard wooden chair, tetchily stubbing out one cigarette and reaching for another, is Sarah. In tie-dye leggings and an army jacket. Talking furiously. About Yeats. And about Scottish history in the Middle Ages. Having two conversations, in fact. One with a friend smoking Woodbines on her left, the other with an American student on her right, whom she has overhead misunderstanding 'An Irish Airman Foresees his Death'. Sentences from one flow into the other and back again. Her listeners struggle to keep up. But she doesn't. 'Why fight for someone else's cause?' 'You've got to remember the Gaelic kings!'

HISTORY

Sarah has history. By descent Irish, by upbringing Catholic, by conviction rebellious. Each aspect builds upon the other. And she is full of stories. From the past she studies, from the novels she reads and from the life she leads. They feed each other, growing in the re-telling. Asked by a history tutor to defend an essay on Mary, Queen of Scots, she leans in and lets fly one line after another, justifying not her essay but the dead queen's actions. It's personal. You sense she was there. Walking beside her. You sense it matters. And really it does. After all, what's the point of talking about it otherwise? 'He gave in,' she tells me, 'after half an hour. He saw my point of view. I got my grade.'

In another class, she has to give a talk on German women between the wars. It's social history. Fresh air after a year of dry political stuff. The tutor is lean and angular, a city person who writes about urban history. She wonders why he is here. His class is well-stocked with Wee Marys – shy Scottish women from Perth, Arbroath and other small towns. They want something new, something that speaks to them. He breathes the fragile world of Weimar Germany into their class. But it is Sarah who gives it life. She watches the films, absorbs them, and seems to embody the 'new woman' of that time. Her hair is shorter. Her clothes more fitted. She has new heroines: Louise Brooks in *Pandora's Box*, Marlene Dietrich in *The Blue Angel*, all the female rowers in *Kuhle Wampe*. But she won't talk well of *Triumph of the Will*. That Leni Riefenstahl – friend of Hitler. She's had enough exposure.

LIVING

Sarah reads. All the time. She starts with the papers over breakfast. In a café. First the sport, then the culture, then the news. She inhales black coffee and cigarettes, followed by a bacon sandwich or the full works. Then, later in the day, she moves on to novels, poetry, biographies. Literary fiction alongside crime stories, alongside romance. The student association bookshop is hopeless. Too small. Stocking class reading lists and not much beside. But there's a better one on Market Street. And they take her cheques, as they bounce from an account straining under the weight of her addiction to literature into the drawer beside the till.

Lunch is with friends. In the Central Bar, a pub near the top of College Street, the last resting post before the trudge to the lecture schools of the arts faculty. Inside, it's thick with undergraduates avoiding the library and a few needy lecturers trying to be their mates. 'All my friends are outsiders here,' she says. Americans, Irish, Catholics, Londoners. But it's not quite true. She makes friends easily. With all sorts. And besides, the true analysis is that we are a lucky, privileged group. Not all the same but all Dionysian in spirit. Here, we have the time and space and freedom to indulge. And we do. We are so cut off. The place is so small. You are never more than ten minutes' walk from fields and farms. You can do all your work and party all you like. You can live like a cavalier and work like a roundhead. Or you can just be the cavalier. There's not much else to do.

Some of us live in St Andrews. Others in big down-at-heel Victorian and Edwardian houses in the Fife countryside, rented out by farmers with better things to do than restore them. Some drive out for weekends. Others come into town for lectures. Town and country; a national way of life lived in miniature, styled out of the past. But with our contemporary taste in music, literature and stimulants. We live under a geodesic dome of indifference to the world outside.

There are parties, lots of them. Sarah is at their heart. Re-making herself at each. Shedding her indie-kid skin for post-war glamour. Coco Chanel and Audrey Hepburn provide the template. At each one, she is wrapped up in conversations, with one person after another. Her art is life. In making the connection. Seeing the interesting part in someone else. And drawing it out. She is an author of reality. Of people becoming themselves. Her characters breathe and talk. They are her friends and all those she meets. She sketches them out better than they know how to themselves.

IRELAND

It's the summer term. St Andrews has a system for its first two years: if you do well in second-term tests, you are exempt from third-term exams. Sarah and I have exemptions. All we have to do is turn up to class occasionally in the first five weeks and turn in essays. It's a system begging to be debauched. And we take full advantage. 'Let's go to Dublin,' she says. 'It's better there.' So we do, crossing Scotland by train to Stranraer and then by ferry to Larne. On the way, Sarah sings rebel songs of 1916 and after. We talk of Edward Carson and James Connolly, Gladstone's Home Rule Bill and De Valera's rectitude, and of the Irish Republican Brotherhood. For us, the past is here, in the present. But we know little of the reality of current life in the north of Ireland. The train from Belfast to Dublin stops near the border. We whisper and wonder if there's a bomb on the line. But the conductor says it's sheep.

In Dublin we stay in a B&B on Upper Gardiner

Street. It's shabby, friendly and cheap. Our host-
ess has cranked open the money box on the pay-
phone in the corridor so she can take out the
50p coins and re-feed them in as she calls family
in America. 'Call who you like,' she says, 'for as
long as you want.' We live off her fried breakfasts
and welcome.

Dublin is what Sarah wanted. There are parts
of her mythology all around. It's a living story and
she is telling it breathlessly as we walk from the
Four Courts to O'Connell Street and then across
the bridge to College Park and Trinity. We have
planned to follow in the footsteps of Bloom and
Dedalus. But we get chest infections and are confined to our room, leaving only to see the doctor
and his cousin the pharmacist. We feed the 50ps
into the phone and call the modern history department to explain our delayed return. 'We are having a reading week.' It's sort of true. Though the
days are spent reading novels from Hodges Figgis,
not course books. On our last day, we take our
sore, wet, bronchial lungs out for the night, grab a
cab and drink cocktails in a room in Temple Bar.

We are triumphant. Dublin almost beat us but in the end it is we who have won.

HORSE RACING

Sarah goes to the races, in the small independent bookies tucked into the side of the faded art nouveau-style Victoria café building. It's a tiny place. Plastic ashtrays brim over on the counter where the slips and pens are found. There cannot be room for more than eight or so people. And they are all men. Middle-aged, in nylon slacks and anoraks. Hair thinning, dentistry indeterminate, with heads cranked upwards on fleshy necks to follow the races on the screen in the far corner. It's a club. It's always been like this. And it's closed to new members.

She pushes the door, it gives and she stumbles in. She has copies of both the *Racing Post* and the *Sporting Life* under her arm. They are her credentials. Unfolding them, she turns to the racecards for the day. There are already crosses by her picks. With a swift hand she completes her slips and breezes to the counter. The men are watching her from the corners of their eyes. They are silent. But then they don't look like talkers. Or winners. Though it's clear the next race will be between them and her.

It's over quickly. From the off there is silence in the room. Except for Sarah, who is muttering nervously about the form. After a minute her voice rises in volume, in pitch. She has an each-way bet and it's looking good. No one else looks hopeful. In the final moments, she splits the room with sound, 'Come on Cuddy Dale!' 'Come on, you beauty!' And then, it's done. The filly has won. The horse placed and there's money for drinks upstairs. No one else moves to the counter. No one else collects. The club has a new member.

JOURNALISM

It's 1994. Towards the end. The future quickens. In the afterlife, Sarah wants to be a journalist. She talks of Martha Gellhorn, Anna Wintour and Julie Burchill. She is in a hurry to get going. But the student paper is to be pitied. Words die on the page, three-dimensional stories are flattened into two and the breath of life is squeezed out from every article, leaving a re-used tea bag in an empty cup. So, we start our own – Sarah, our friend James and I. Other friends pitch in. We've no clue. No money. No advertising. And no distribution. But we have Sarah and her liquid, distilled, 100 per cent proof enthusiasm. It will be great. And it is. Sort of. A mix of comment, culture and surreal humour. Not polished, not perfect but a triumph of the will. Her will.

It doesn't last. But for one moment, the veil of St Andrews' reality has a tear in it. Through it, you can glimpse who she will become. Later, Sarah will learn her craft. After St Andrews, there is a scholarship to go to America to study journalism at NYU. And after that, the subbing and writing on shifts in London and Manchester, where she will learn all over again. But it was in a café in a small town on Scotland's east coast where her eyes brightened and the words flowed as she set out what she was going to do and who she was going to be.

Scars

SOME EVENINGS, WHEN I AM FEELING PARTICULARLY SELF-LOATHING, I TAKE ALL MY CLOTHES OFF AND STAND NAKED IN THE BATHROOM STUDYING THE WAYS IN WHICH MY BODY HAS CHANGED.

I look at the hollows round my collar bone and the shadows under my eyes. I peer in the mirror to see if my eyes have become more or less yellow, an aspect of having pseudo-cirrhosis that can only worsen as my liver continues to fail.

I stare at my withered breasts, both the real one and the fake one. The latter was so beautifully plump when it was first built, now it has sunk in on itself as my disease has progressed.

I examine the alien in the mirror – the bald head, the sparse eyelashes, the barely there eyebrows – because it is impossible to look away.

My body marks the way in which the disease is progressing through me and, deep inside me, an almost atavistic need pulses, whispering: 'Bear witness to this.'

The event that caused the first scar I can remember getting occurred when I was seven years old. Like all traumatic memories, the moment it happened is burned deep within me and the events seem to unfold in vivid, so-bright-it-hurts colours.

It was early evening, after school. My mother was still at work and we were being looked after by a childminder, who was busy with my younger brother in another part of the house. My younger sister and I were sprawled in the TV room watching *Dogtanian and The Three Muskehounds*, and the cartoon dogs on TV made me think affectionately of our own dog, a somewhat irascible beagle named Humphrey, whom we had had for a couple of months and who was currently curled up on the chair next to mine.

You can probably see where this is going . . .

I climbed onto the chair with Humphrey and woke him by giving him a hug. Unfortunately, not only had I woken him up but I had the temerity to be sitting in my mother's chair. Beagles are pack dogs and Humphrey was slavishly loyal to my mother. Before I could move away, he snarled, turned and bit me on the leg.

Shocked, I hit him, causing him to jump off the chair and curl up in a different part of the room. 'Poor Humphrey,' said my sister as, still in shock, I stared down at the blood dripping from my leg onto the floor.

Eventually, my sister would snap into action and call the childminder. She would get hold of my mum and I would end up getting seven stiches in hospital. The subsequent scar is a white, raised mark on my inner thigh. Every time that I look at it I am reminded that you don't always have to do something with malicious intent; sometimes simply failing to think through the consequences of your actions will extract a price.

As for Humphrey, two weeks later he nipped my little brother, still a toddler, on the lip when he bent in to kiss him and was subsequently rehoused with an elderly lady who kept another beagle and was used to them. We did not get another dog.

(Humphrey's fate has long been a source of contention between my sister and me. She insists he was put down and our parents lied to us. I am adamant that they told the truth. My mother has always claimed that I am correct and given that both my sister and I are now in our forties, I see no reason for her to be lying.)

My mastectomy scar is an absence rather than presence. When I look in the mirror I see not a disfiguring line or raised mark but rather a circle where my nipple should be. It wasn't supposed to be like this.

When the removal and reconstruction of my left breast took place the plan was straightforward.

I would finish my radiation treatment, lose a bit of weight and then my wonderful plastic surgeon would add my nipple and reduce and lift my right breast so that it was in line with the newly perky left one. But my cancer's sudden return and rapid spread meant that these plans were halted, leaving me with a saggy and droopy breast on my right side and a left breast with a circular scar where once I expected a perfect nipple to be.

From ribs to kidneys, there are many body parts you never really think about until you hurt them or something starts to go wrong. For me, nipples fell under that category. They were just appendages on the end of breast, occasionally sucked by those I went to bed with and more firmly attacked by my two children as babies, both of whom had an extremely firm clamp.

If the birth of my children reminded me of their existence, the stillbirth that followed served a bitter message about nurture and nature as my baby died but my milk continued to come in.

I lay in hospital in New York crying about my

lost baby while a series of well-intentioned lactation specialists tried to get me to express the milk that was painfully building up. I did as they told me but all I could think was that my baby should be there, greedily gulping and draining me dry in ten minutes just as the other two did.

A decade later, I would stand in the bathroom, stare at the space where my nipple once was and think: Yes, this is terrible. Yes I look awful. But nothing will ever feel quite as awful as those nights of wild, untrammelled grief when all I wanted was to wake up and find my daughter miraculously alive and crying to be fed in that mewing, half-helpless way so many newborns do.

My second set of scars are a series of faded white lines running up my right arm. They come into sharp focus only when I tan and are a bitter remembrance of a period of my life when I felt overwhelmed with emotion and out of control.

In the miserable year I spent at a very posh co-educational Edinburgh private school, known for educating future prime ministers and fictional spies, I knew a lot of girls who self-harmed. Astonishingly, most of them were boarders (I was a day pupil) and yet their housemistress seemed barely aware that her toilets were full of unhappy young women scraping razors down their arms. Fascinated, I would watch as they dressed their cuts, wondering what exactly they achieved when they hurt themselves in this way. It was only a matter of time before I joined them.

I cannot speak for my fellow pupils, some of whom would turn out to have serious and long-standing depression, but for me cutting provided release. Release from the maelstrom of emotion that regularly threatened to overwhelm me. Release from my fast-burning temper. Release from moments where everything seemed just too much and I felt entirely out of control.

At the time, such actions seemed momentous. I would look at the blood welling from the shallow cuts on my arm and feel a sense of calm. Now everything would be under control, I would think. I don't have a problem, I just feel too much.

Ah, the self-involved arrogance of the teenage mind.

In reality, I was only ever playing at self-harm. Once my hormones had settled, my emotions regulated and, crucially, once I left the toxic environment of that particular school, I stopped feeling the need to regularly cut myself. By the time I went to university two years later I had stopped all together.

These days the scars are only faintly visible and when I look at them the emotion I feel most strongly is shame. Shame at the way in which I thought I should join those others girls rather than being a good friend and trying to help them or seeking help for them; shame at my spoiled privilege which led me to essentially appropriate other people's harmful coping mechanisms as my own; shame at the attention seeking, the acting out, the denial about the path I was taking and, most of all, shame that I never told my parents, to whom I had always been close, about what I was doing or how very unhappy I was at that school, preferring instead to push at the boundaries until I was essentially asked to leave.

There is, however, one thing that I have no shame about at all and that is the emotions I felt at that time, something my sister, who sees similar traits in her oldest daughter, describes as having 'all the feels'. Teenagers should feel things strongly. They should laugh hard and cry hard and hurl themselves at life. I cannot deny that I acted foolishly as an overwrought teen but occasionally, when I look at those white lines, it isn't shame I feel but an odd acceptance that things might not always have been great but, even at that terrible school, there were still moments when I laughed so much with friends that I became entirely incapable of speech.

My port-a-cath lies just below my skin. Sometimes it looks as though it might pop out altogether. Its purpose is to allow easy access for everything from chemotherapy to bloods – in practice, things aren't always quite as straightforward.

I have always had bad veins. They sit very deep under my skin, are hard to access and prone to collapse. When I first moved to New York as a student one of my visa requirements was a negative AIDS test for which I had to give blood. Pretty much every vein in both arms was blown out before they finally managed to get blood (painfully) from a vein in my foot.

Similarly, at Queen Charlotte's Hospital in Hammersmith, I used to squeak and shout so often that Kris would have to tell the other expectant mothers: 'Don't worry, she just has really bad veins.' Things improved when we moved to New York where the doctors took one look at my arms and ensured that all my bloods were taken by the phlebotomists.

The port should have helped with these problems and it largely did. However, the first I had fitted was inserted far too deep 'for cosmetic reasons'. This despite the fact that I couldn't have cared less about whether you could see the port and wasn't even consulted about my wishes. It was hard to access – even highly experienced chemo nurses struggled – and I frequently ended up asking them to use a needle instead. I had it removed during my mastectomy.

Unfortunately, I also had 27 lymph nodes removed from my left arm at the same time. This meant that when my cancer returned six weeks later and I had another port fitted (this one mercifully near the surface and thus easy to access) I could no longer have anyone draw blood through my left arms for fear of giving me lymphoedema*, always the one thing I knew I truly could not bear. You might be thinking at this moment: 'But surely the re-fitting of the port meant that this did not matter?' Unfortunately, the port cannot be used for everything. There were fluids to be given at the same time as blood transfusions; scans where protocol stated the port shouldn't be used; emergency admissions to non-chemo wards where they weren't sure how to use the port so used the veins instead; a surgical procedure where the sedative could not be administered through the port. All of this means that my crumbling veins continue to be prodded and poked. They still frequently collapse. They often blow out. But it happens less frequently than before thanks to

---

* Irreversible swelling in limbs due to lack of lymph nodes.

that port pulsing beneath my skin, serving a welcome and often much-needed reminder that not every scar is a hurtful, painful one.

❧

Not every scar is a serious one. Some are reminders of giggling nights when accidents happened and were easily laughed away the next morning. I have torn a ligament wearing a ridiculous pair of high heels while stumbling arm-in-arm down the cobbled streets of Edinburgh's Old Town; dented my head and given myself two black eyes just before starting a journalism traineeship after exuberantly swinging around a concrete lamppost following a slightly too-enjoyable day watching Euro '96 and managed to gouge a hole in my leg after tripping over my clothes horse in heels following a raucous dinner party (rather too many of my early-to-late twenties scars involve a lethal combination of high heels and drink. I grew out of it).

The scar that makes me laugh the most thinking back is the summer I broke my toe. Not because breaking your little toe is in anyway funny but because of the circumstances under which it happened. A close friend and her brother had come to stay with us and her brother developed a big crush on my little sister. Unfortunately, the crush was not reciprocated and she spent the evening kissing someone else instead.

The next day, that boy rang and my friend's brother dashed to the phone to claim that my sister wasn't in. Desperate to stop him from insulting the caller, I ran to grab the phone from his hand and in doing so whacked my little toe across a metal bar. I wasn't wearing shoes and the pain was excruciating. Looking down, I could see my toe didn't look right in any way. 'I think I may have broken it,' I said, before laughing at the stupidity of the situation.

My mother told me to head to my dad's surgical clinic, where he pointed out he hadn't set toes for years, so I did the sensible thing and waited in A&E to have it fixed. I spent the rest of the summer with my left foot wrapped in a bandage and enchased in a blue plastic shoe, hopping around like a pirate queen who has lost her tribe.

It was such a silly injury sustained in such a silly way and, while it hurt like hell at the time, these days the images that cling to my mind are that desperate over-the-top tussle for the phone (which now feels almost like something from a bad teen movie) and the memory of hopping around everywhere and trying not to overbalance and fall.

They are memories of a lighter, more silly time and when I think of them I cannot help but laugh.

Nor is every scar always visible. When the cancer moved to my liver it stopped being a tangible thing I could touch, a solid lump that I could feel – and feel reducing. Instead, it spread, as my oncologist evocatively said, like a series of speckled eggs or freckles, dots across the whole of the liver rather than one solid tumour. I cried when I first learned about those dots, cried because there would be no easy option but instead more rounds of chemo, until it stopped working and I died.

Yet those tears didn't last for long. I thought about the situation and decided that, while acknowledging it and accepting that it wasn't the best or easiest of hands to have been dealt, the only way to get through it was to take positives from every day: I was alive, I could work. I spent time with Kris, my children and the dog; I took as much enjoyment as I could out of the day; and looked only forward, never down at the vertiginous chasm lurking below, waiting to swallow me whole – and crucially never back at what could have been but wasn't.

So began round after round of chemotherapy, blasting the liver and miraculously keeping the tumours there rather than letting them spread. There were setbacks, too, however. Chief among them was discovering that capecitabine, the commonly used and often very effective oral chemotherapy, didn't hold my tumour in place – instead, while on it, the tumours, which had been reduced, vigorously returned.

At which point I decided to try Sirtex, an experimental treatment in which the tumours are blasted with radiotherapy, attacking and reducing them. It was reputedly painful and had some side effects, most notably its long-term effects on the liver. But I thought it was worth the shot. I was also extremely lucky because my husband held private healthcare and Sirtex is difficult to wrangle on the NHS.

They were right, too, that the procedure was painful, particularly so as I turned out to have two arterial entrances on one side of my liver, which made it harder to get the radiotherapy in. Sore as it was it worked, hitting every part of the tumour and reducing it considerably.

It was not, however, without side effects. My liver struggled to cope with the ongoing chemo and began to become cirrhotic. I developed ascites, a liquid build-up in the abdomen which made life more difficult as the pain increased. Much of this would have happened anyway – there was only so long that the liver and chemo could stay in balance, particularly given the aggression of my tumour – but the Sirtex potentially sped up the process.

Not that I regret it. It reduced my tumour and helped keep me alive. Like most things connected to my liver, its effects remain invisible, scars that can be neither felt nor seen, but sometimes I lie in bed at night imagining it erasing all those tumour freckles only for them to return, ready for battle once more.

❧

Some scars bring both joy and sorrow. I have had three C-sections: the first two gave me my children, Ruby and Oisín, the third delivered my stillborn daughter Iris. When I look at these scars in the mirror, it reminds me how powerful the human body can be, bringing both life and death into the world.

When Kris and I moved to New York, I was six months pregnant with Ruby. Close friends and relative strangers all warned us that giving birth in America was a highly medicalised experience, that I was almost certain to end up trapped in a hospital bed and having a C-section. As a fairly pragmatic person, I shrugged away such concerns: a birth is a birth, it doesn't matter how you deliver the baby and in the UK far too much time is given to the notion of the perfect mother with the perfect birth plan, whose perfect delivery means that they bond more easily with their child because they weren't 'too posh to push'.

Despite that being a load of nonsense, it is true that the US system leans too much the other way, can be high risk given surgery is so often involved and is exorbitant for those without medical insurance – something we thankfully had because of Kris's relocation work package.

Almost from the beginning it was inevitable how this pregnancy would evolve. My family has a history of late births and at almost 40 weeks, Ruby showed no signs of arriving. An induction was planned. Then my waters broke but I didn't go into labour. In the UK they would tell you to stay at home until labour began but my New York hospital had different ideas.

I was told to come in, put in a bed and given a cocktail of drugs to help the process along. By 2am the next night, I still wasn't in full labour but Ruby had moved down and it was inevitable that she would be delivered by C-section, particularly because my gynaecologist was simultaneously dealing with a far more high-risk and complicated pregnancy in the next room. I was wheeled to surgery where 30 minutes later my daughter arrived and I promptly threw up over the anaesthetist, who took it remarkably well.

Oisín's birth was more straightforward. Having no family in New York and with a two-year-old to be cared for, an elective C-section seemed the obvious solution. The procedure took half an hour and I felt rather like a washing machine with a baby being pulled out instead of clothes. In the end, it was probably just as well that we opted for the operation as my son was a large baby who essentially looked like a jolly Russian sailor or a mob boss built on the Tony Soprano scale.

When I look at those faint scars in the mirror late at night it brings back all the joy and fear and sheer intensity of giving birth. I look at them and feel a wave of happiness – these scars came from bringing my children into the world and I will never understand those whose immediate desire is to remove them, to eradicate any trace of imperfection from their bodies. To my mind, your body is a map made up of hard-won experiences and its scars should serve as both acknowledgement and celebration of that fact.

That remains true even when the scar brings sorrow, as it does for me with Iris. I had the option to be unconscious during her delivery but couldn't take it. If I had been awake for my two live pregnancies I couldn't abandon my dead daughter by sleeping through her birth. It was hard. I wept throughout and barely remember most of it, bar the moments I held her tiny body and cried and sang the songs that I sang to Ruby and Oisín to help them sleep at night.

Yet now, when so much else has happened, and so many other scars cross my body, I can look at the scar from Iris's birth with different eyes. My body can deliver both life and death. There is something very powerful about that. It may be devastating but it is also a reminder that while we cannot control every circumstance what we can do is acknowledge that there is a quiet strength in accepting that and letting the darkness in.

The scar that has caused the most trouble and the one I despair of is that of my ascitic drain. For two years my cancer was held in place and even reduced by various chemotherapy treatments but then in March 2020, just as Covid-19 and the lockdown occurred, my liver finally said enough and I developed ascites. After testing, the ascites turned out not to be malignant or cancer-related but rather a result of all the treatments, which had essentially given me cirrhosis. Because of the pandemic, I was initially given a series of temporary drains with the hope that regular draining would relieve the issue and reduce the problem. Unfortunately, this turned out not to be the case. Instead, the fluid continued to build and the draining seemed to have little effect. In September, the decision was taken to put in a permanent drain.

At first, everything was pretty straightforward. The procedure was easy, despite my squeamishness about needles and local anaesthetic in particular. The drain was not uncomfortable and Kris was fantastic at cleaning the dressing and helping me regularly drain at home. At which point everything that could possibly go wrong did.

I began to develop infections, each one more resistant than the last. I went back and forth between hospital and home, and spent my time feeling either exhausted or invigorated, a situation that was far more tiring then it might seem.

Increasingly worried about the infections, my failing liver and the issues with recovery, the medical team decided to remove the initial drain and insert a new one on my left side instead. Again, this all went very smoothly. Two weeks later, it all fell apart. Another infection. This one even more resistant to treatment. It not only saw me back in hospital but also coincided with a collapse in my leg muscles driven by the fluid build-up.

In a frustratingly short period, I went from cooking, writing and moving around with ease to wobbling around like a woman decades older with my legs constantly giving way. The doctors decided not to remove this drain because they'd simply have to insert another and the infections were likely to continue. Instead, the only thing we could do was walk the tightrope and try to get the balance right between the liver and the cancer treatment, a near impossible task. It was a depressing turn of events and one that meant that Kris and I now had to consider full-time care and the fact that time was almost certainly running out.

This is where things currently stand. I can't deny that of all my scars, it is the hole where the drain is that I loathe the most. It's hard to love something that you link with the probable end of your life and harder still when you remember that prior to its existence, and even in the early days of its insertion, life continued as normally as it could. In my more realistic moments, I recognise that this decline was inevitable – all the talk about fighting or beating cancer being a load of hooey, cancer kills and 31 people die every day from metastatic breast cancer – but I still can't help but loathe and blame the drain.

For not all scars are created equally. There are those that make you laugh and those which you can barely stand to see. My drain scar is the latter and for all that it prolonged my life, it also brought my death into focus. That's a hard thing to grapple with, let alone embrace each day.

∽

Standing naked in front of the mirror in my bathroom this is what I see: a skinny, yellowing body with little hair, swollen legs and a distended stomach. Sometimes I feel as though I look like the alien Mekon of Mekonta from the old *Dan Dare* comics my grandfather gave us to read over long childhood summers in Bournemouth. Other times, as though I am a newly hatched fledgling, a baby bird who cannot fly to safety and good health but will instead plummet squawking onto the cold, hard ground.

Most of all, however, I see those scars. My new breast once plump and beautiful, now sagging like the rest of me; the tiny dimple where my port lives; the C-sections that cross my abdomen; the dog bite on my inner thigh. I see the shallow white lines on my right arm and the faint line on my toe. I glance down at the hole on my right side where the first drain lived and at the one on my right where the new drain is positioned. I look at these scars, both loved and hated, and see them for what they are: trophies.

The marks that I bear on my body are a testimony to my life, a living map of all that I have been through, both good and bad. It is for this reason that I can embrace even the worst of them – because they are part of me. They tell the story of my life, both the good moments and the bad. And because of that they are a comfort, a reminder that you may not be able to see the future but that doesn't mean that you can't enjoy what's left of life. Because despite everything – the endless treatments, the setbacks, the infections, the constant trips to hospital, the prodding and poking and loss of dignity of the past two years – so much pleasure has been available to me as well.

From family holidays to simply lying around with Kris and the kids, playing games, watching TV together, chatting with my sister and close friends, laughing at our crazy but loving dog, I have embraced it all. In the same way I embrace my scars. They are part of me as yours are a part of you, and it is far better to acknowledge and try to love them then it is to flinch and look away.

How Cancer Gave Me Back My Sense of Fashion

IT WAS WHEN I OPENED MY WARDROBE AND SAW A SEEMINGLY ENDLESS LINE OF SUMMER DRESSES, IN EVERY PATTERN AND HUE FROM PALEST PINK TO BRIGHT YELLOW, BLACK AND COVERED IN ROSES, WHITE WITH CHERRIES PRINTED ON, SHORT, MIDI AND FULL LENGTH, MANY YET TO BE WORN, THAT I REAL-ISED I MIGHT JUST HAVE A SHOPPING PROBLEM. The combination of cancer and Covid pandemic had fuelled my desire to look if not good then at least stylish, even if circumstances meant that no one apart from Kris and the kids would really see. Throw a sudden dramatic weight loss into the mix, which meant that for the first time in years I could actually wear the little flippy dresses from France I so enjoyed looking at on various websites, and you had the seeds for what was turning out to be an unstoppable addiction.

Most importantly, it was the first time that I had truly cared about looking good in years – in fact, a recent trawl through old photographs had embarrassingly suggested that I had pretty much worn the same dress most days for five years, after which it fell apart – which meant that I could honestly say, forget makeovers and fashion shows, flicking through fashion magazines or wasting time on Instagram, it took stage IV cancer to make me fall in love with fashion once again.

It wasn't always this way. In my teens and twenties, I had a keen interest in fashion. Growing up in Edinburgh, itself a dark and gothic city, it made sense to be a goth myself and thus I had the obligatory backcombed hair, fishnet tights and black skirts, usually worn with a Sisters of Mercy or The Mission band t-shirt. The brief trend for Americana led to the purchase of a baseball jacket of which I was inordinately proud. The rest of the time, I tended to slope around in black cardigans and black dresses with the occasional splash of purple thrown in.

As we got older, so indie became more popular. I clomped around in a series of short skirts, Doc Marten boots, an army shirt and the obligatory band t-shirt, most usually The Pixies or Nirvana, occasionally Dinosaur Jr. or Mudhoney instead.

Then came university and my first encounter with one of the best books about fashion ever written: Lee Tulloch's *Fabulous Nobodies*, in which her heroine, the wonderfully named Reality Nirvana Tuttle, works as a 'doorwhore' for a New York nightclub and names all her clothes, which she talks to, after famous Hollywood stars.

Inspired by Tulloch's genius, I realised that fashion didn't have to be all about following rules or looking chic – it could be an exercise in dressing up and trying out different personas. There were days when I woke up and felt like Sonic Youth's Kim Gordon, which meant pulling on jeans and a band t-shirt, throwing on my leopard print coat and a beanie hat and pretending that I spent my time practising to become famous with my imaginary Seattle band.

Then there were days when I felt more like a lost female member of the Manic Street Preachers, which meant wearing my vintage lambswool jacket with fake fur collar or the leopard print coat once again, this time with fishnet tights, Doc Marten boots and the shortest of mini-skirts: two that I was particularly fond of were a button-through tiger print and an iridescent blue skirt made of a strange plastic material. Both had been bought in Kensington Market's Sign of the Times.

I had a tartan bondage dress for when I was feeling more dressy and a babydoll halterneck which I wore when I felt like cos-playing as Hole singer Courtney Love. There were Stussy shirts and t-shirts for the moments when I felt like a skater girl and the obligatory Adidas Gazelles that no self-respecting Britpop fan could be without.

There were trips to Glasgow where I bought black mohair jumpers along with the week's new releases, while back home in London I read and reread *Edie: An American Biography* by Jean Stein, which details the sad, short and chic life of Andy Warhol's most famous muse, and scoured vintage shops buying pretty blouses and a pink tweed suit. Not for me the monotony of trench coats, little neck scarfs, perfectly cut jeans and sticking to a look.

Like Reality, I felt as though I had 57 fashion personas and every morning might birth a different, more exciting one.

This belief in the transformative power of clothes continued throughout my twenties. I moved with my then boyfriend Adrian to Berlin for three months, during which I spent my money on a series of mini-skirts and Sixties-style faux tweed coats from Kookai, had my hair cut into a sharp, dark red bob and wore knee-high boots. None of this was particularly practical in Berlin in January. Indeed, it was so cold that one day even my eyelashes froze and Adrian suggested that I might be better off wrapping up against the cold rather than sliding down the icy streets wearing a flimsy coat and beret.

I shrugged him off. Suffering was a well-known side effect of looking stylish, I informed him. To his credit, he managed not to laugh directly at me, although there might have been a silent snort as I left our tiny room in Wilmersdorf. Undeterred by his amusement, I would trudge through the snow to the local English language cinema, trying not to slip in my high-heeled boots and pretending that I was a spy from a John Le Carré novel or Emma Peel in *The Avengers*.

Back in London, I bought a beautiful moss green tweed suit from Gerard Darel, which I thought of as my French lesbian's suit because it seemed like the sort of thing a 1930s lesbian French detective might wear. No, I don't know how I decided this, it's simply how it was. I wore it with a crisp white shirt from Agnès B. and felt as though, for the first time in my life, I might be managing to pull off chic rather than simply experimenting with style.

I bought another tweed skirt as well, longer and cut on the bias, which I would wear with a vintage grey collared top and a string of pearls. While I loved the look it wasn't entirely successful: when

I wore it to a 1996 march against the Major government's cuts, Adrian told me that he felt he was going to a protest with a Mitford sister. He didn't intend it as a compliment but I smiled anyway.

❧

Then in 1997, just as Britain elected Tony Blair to power, I won a scholarship to New York University to study for a journalism MA and my whole world changed. Here was the high fashion, low trash city of my dreams. I was in Reality Tuttle's stalking ground, where surely all my fashion dreams would come true.

I knew within days that I didn't actually want to be a fashion journalist (my interest at that time lay in covering sport and features and I was lucky enough to be taught the latter by the great feminist pop critic and feature writer Ellen Willis). I had no desire to work for Condé Nast or submit myself to the icy glare of Anna 'Nuclear' Wintour but I did want to search every second-hand shop and every independent boutique in the city.

As a student, I didn't have much money but

the mid-1990s was a time when people could still both live and thrive in the city. Gentrification had yet to really happen and the Village, where my university was, had plenty of cheap places to eat, including Veselka, a 24-hour Ukrainian diner which made pierogi to die for, and Kiev, where Allen Ginsberg and Quentin Crisp were among the famous regulars.

It was also full of the most incredible shops. On Eighth Street I found a shoe shop that made the sort of one-of-a-kind shoes that make people stop in the street and stare. I spent a month saving up for a pair of sandals with an intricately carved wooden five-inch platform held in place by a similarly intricate wooden ball. I have them still and on the rare occasions when I wear them strangers still stop me to tell me how fabulous they are.

I discovered Betsey Johnson and bought sparkling cardigans and little floral dresses. I spent happy weekends travelling out to Brooklyn and rooting through the rails of charity shops before heading back to Manhattan to root around the vintage shops in St Mark's Place or hang out at the

Canal Jean Co where you could buy both vintage and new jackets and jeans.

New York was slowly changing but it still felt like a place where anyone could make it, provided you had a little bit of pizzazz and a willingness to stand out from the crowd. In the yet-to-be-gentrified Meatpacking District I would sit at late-night cafés and try not to stare at the flamboyant transgender women walking past; at Marie's Crisis Café I would listen as incredible performers sang showtunes in a tiny piano bar, tapping those wooden platforms against the floor and trying out every look from vintage wiggle dresses to tiny mini-skirts and patent knee-high boots.

Sadly, even the best of times must come to end, and in 1999 I moved back to the UK, where a series of events conspired to ensure that I lost my fashion mojo for almost two decades.

It didn't happen overnight. In fact, I initially tried quite hard to stay fashionable, spending money on stylish shoes from Kurt Geiger and suits from

Jesire, French Connection and, memorably, in a sale, a Prada dress and suit. Then, at the beginning of the new century, I moved to Manchester to work at the *Manchester Evening News*. I was living alone, working from 8am until 4pm and filling my free hours with trips to the pub and pizza. Inevitably, I put on weight.

That weight gain didn't instantly stop my interest in fashion but there was a slow but sure tailing off. I loved my job as a feature writer and was determined to do well at it. This meant working long hours, which in turn meant that I cared less about my physical appearance and more about how the many and varied articles I was writing (I covered everything from the 2002 marches against the Iraq war to a hard-to-get interview with the Gallagher brothers' mum Peggy) were received.

It didn't help that Manchester was the sort of place where people dressed up to the nines complete with immaculate make-up and perfectly put together outfits. I remember going out one night and realising that my friend Alexa and I were the only two women not wearing silk parachute trousers, a strappy top and heels.

In previous times, I would have taken that as a challenge and laughed at the way everyone was following a dress code but the combination of weight gain and being in a new city meant that instead I felt insecure about the situation. Perhaps I should be wearing a similar outfit? Or, if not, then should I at least have attempted to spend more time getting ready? To have applied more make-up? Put some more effort into my hair and outfit?

The more time I spent in Manchester the less inclined I was to do so. Suddenly, fashion and dressing in style seemed like a huge effort. Far easier to opt out and dress down than try to fit in and get it wrong.

The trouble with embracing certain mindsets is that the longer you follow them the harder it is to snap out and move on. I moved back to London but found myself no more inspired than before. Instead, I began working as a sub editor at the *Observer* newspaper while picking up shifts elsewhere. My main shift was on a Saturday and I lived in jeans and jumpers, got my head down and tried not to make too many mistakes when putting my copy through.

It would be easy to presume that I was depressed and that my lack of interest in looking good was connected to this. Actually, the opposite was true. While I did put on weight during this period and while that weight gain made me less interested in clothes, this was also one of the happiest times of my life. It was the time when Kris and I began to go out (we had known each other for a while but the timing had never been right before); an era filled with long nights out, trips abroad to Italy and Spain and endless meals out. I was blissfully happy; perhaps it is fair to say too happy to care about how I looked or how other people might see me.

In November 2006, Kris and I were married. In an attempt to pay lip service to the notion of losing weight ahead of the wedding, I had booked a personal trainer but, in an echo of my similarly half-hearted attempts to learn to drive when at school, I spent more time talking to them then actually working out. Despite this, I still believed that I was going to miraculously lose weight and, partially because of that, I didn't buy my wedding dress until a couple of weeks before the wedding.

It was from Jenny Packham, a short dress which fell to the knee and was covered in intricate beading with a neckline that made the most of my cleavage.

I wore it with red mohair Louboutin shoes – much to the surprise of some of the congregation at the Catholic church where we married – my hair up and as big as it could be and threw a leopard print coat over the top when it came time to leave. Not for me the tasteful, understated wedding: if you can't channel your inner barmaid on your wedding day then frankly there's no point to getting married at all.

Within a year, Kris and I had moved to New York and I was pregnant with our first child. At first, I thought that this would be the opportunity I'd been searching for, a chance to reconnect with my fashion dreams. But it quickly transpired that New York had changed in the past decade – and so had I.

Whereas the city in the mid-1990s still had room for dreamers and those with more flash than cash, it was now a post-*Sex and the City* world. Designer labels were everything; New York women were immaculately put together and without money you couldn't possibly live in Manhattan. It didn't help that I had never liked the popular US comedy, failing to identify with any of the women at its heart, largely because to me, they represented a certain soul-crushing Upper East Side corporateness, a takeover of the wealthy which at best left no room for imagination and risk-taking and at worst forced people out to the margins of their own city, and eventually out of the city all together.

Kris and I settled in Brooklyn where, thanks to his work deal, we had a lovely flat with an understanding landlord and a small backyard. It was a long, hot summer and I lived in maternity clothes and little tea dresses that covered the growing bump.

So far, so normal. The problems came after Ruby was born when I found that I lacked the energy to change the way in which I had dressed for the past nine months. Friends advised me otherwise – I was told it was important to buy a non-maternity dress, something that would make me feel stylish again. The trouble was I simply couldn't be bothered. The little flippy dresses were easy and undemanding, you could throw them on and get on with your day and, best of all, they provided easy access for breastfeeding, meaning that there was little need to rummage around getting into the best position.

To say that I lived in them is something of an understatement: looking back over photographs from the five years we were in New York, a period during which I gave birth to two children and suffered through a stillbirth, I didn't just wear a similar style for five years, I essentially wore the same dress. Sure, occasionally I threw another dress into the mix, while that one was in the wash – I might be untidy and unbothered by fashion but I wasn't an animal – but it seems that I was happy simply to wear the same thing day after day after day. Making it worse was the fact that it was a pretty nondescript dress. It had originally belonged to my sister, had a fairly boring pattern and was a sludgy mix of green and blue. My main reason for repeatedly wearing it was adaptability: it was the sort of dress that you could stick a long sleeve t-shirt under in winter and wear bare armed in the summer heat.

It was around this time too that my friend Tara, who worked in the local wine shop, introduced herself to me by telling me that the way I dressed combined with my hair reminded her of Helena Bonham Carter. Given that I was surrounded by immaculately turned out Brooklyn mothers who hadn't lapsed into throwing cardigans over tea dresses while failing to brush their hair, but who instead wore the universal wardrobe of yummy mummies on both sides of the Atlantic – inky jeans, polo necks, gilets, smart dresses from Banana Republic or J Crew – I began to feel a little concerned.

Not concerned enough to change the way in which I dressed, however. Instead, it would take a move back over the Atlantic and a stage IV cancer diagnosis to help me rediscover my sense of style.

❧

Say to anyone that cancer gave you back your fashion sense and they are likely to raise an eyebrow at the very least. Yet in my case, it's true. Prior to my stage IV diagnosis I had lost all interest in fashion, since it I have existed in a near-permanent shopping state of mind.

That's not to say that it was as simple as getting the diagnosis, waking up the next day and thinking, 'Ah, I have a passion for fashion once more.' Instead, it's more that just as a small series of steps led me to lose all interest in what I wore, so a different series of steps gradually led to a reawakened interest in style.

The first of those steps came during my initial cancer diagnosis: when you start losing all your hair then it is perhaps inevitable that you start to focus more on how you look. When I was healthy I had the luxury of being able to say, 'Oh, it doesn't matter how people see me,' but once I was sick then I began to care more about the image I put forth to the world.

I found that the wigs offered to cancer patients, while impressively realistic to look at, made my head itch too much in the summer (it didn't help that the summer of 2018 was particularly hot and glorious, which made them all the more itchy). Instead, I decided to channel my inner 'younger wife of a Middle Eastern potentate' with a series of dramatic turbans and full-skirted, three-quarter sleeve dresses.

After my mastectomy, my hair began to grow back, thick and curly with a streak of white at the front that I was rather attached to. My post-cancer plan involved a breast reduction and I had been advised to lose some weight before it. Deciding that 46 was an age at which to start taking people seriously when they suggested making a concerted effort to lose weight, I was about to begin when I received the terrible news that my cancer had spread to my liver and was now metastatic.

What followed was a particularly gruelling time when fashion was once again far from my mind. I was on a huge amount of steroids and can barely bring myself to look at photographs from this period: I am hugely fat and bloated with a moon face. I am unrecognisable. I would lie in bed at night and wonder how Kris was able to bring himself to touch me. Having managed to feel positive for large parts of my diagnosis, even the announcement that it had spread, I found myself teetering on the edge of serious depression.

Even now, I'm not sure how that would have played out and I am thankful that I don't have to think about it. For, soon after my worst moment, an otherwise lovely trip to Edinburgh with my brother and sister that was almost ruined when I looked back over the photographs and realised how enormous and unwell I appeared, my oncologist took me off the steroids. The effects were almost immediate. The weight slid from my face and body. I stopped looking bloated and became more of a normal size.

More unusually, the weight continued to fall off, partially because it was then that I developed ascites, which required regular draining, and partially because of the cancer's progression. It was at this point that a small voice in my head noted that this was not necessarily a good thing. It was drowned out, however, by a louder voice that acknowledged that even so, it was actually quite nice not to be overweight for the first time in almost two decades.

At this point, I was definitely moving into tricky waters. It is one thing to want to be stylish and quite another to equate style with being a certain weight. We are repeatedly warned against patholo-gizing how we look, believing that looking one way is good and another is bad. Yet I would be lying if I didn't admit that there was a certain satisfac-tion in watching my weight initially drop and then stabilise. It is worth noting that this was a weight loss caused by sickness; at no point did I restrict my food or diet. I ate healthily, as encouraged by the nutritionist, but I also didn't deny myself cer-tain foods if I wanted them and was at one point ordered to drink whole milk and eat cheese for pro-tein purposes.

Most importantly, from my personal view-point, the most exciting thing about the end of the body bloating and moon face was the new oppor-tunities to wear different clothes. After a couple of years of feeling deeply uncomfortable about how

I looked and spending my time dreaming about fashion rather than wearing it, suddenly I could make those dreams come true.

Prior to this, I had fantasised about clothes rather than buying them. I embraced the concept of imaginary fashion; that is, whole outfits that existed in my head rather than in real life. There were days when I was Margaret Howell Woman, wearing guernseys, immaculate shirts and perfectly cut navy trousers and staring out to sea from the potter's cottage in which I lived (no, I don't know why Margaret Howell Woman was a potter but in my mind she/I always was). Or I was living in Paris during the Belle Epoque, where I spent my time with Romaine Brooks and Natalie Barney, wearing sharp men's tailoring, or in Devon's 'Hangover Hall' in the 1930s, watching Djuna Barnes complete *Nightwood*.

I was Mitford sister and Biba girl; I queued for Dior's New Look and joined the hordes thronging outside The Limelight, CBGBs and Studio 54. I was nightclub star and dolly bird, rocker and mod, punk and post-punk and indie queen. Gina Lollobrigida strutting down the Via del Corso and

Katharine Hepburn setting a new trend with the sharpest of slacks.

But only ever in my dreams.

Now, suddenly and surprisingly, thanks to a combination of long-saved money and weight loss, I had the opportunity to act on those impulses. I could shop at French boutiques such as Rouje, stocking up on their Gabin dresses and lipsticks in every possible shade of red. I could buy perfectly cut jumpers from Navygrey and Me+Em and full skirts from Uniqlo, Whistles and Collectif.

I rummaged through online vintage shops such as the Seamstress of Bloomsbury and browsed the shirt dresses at ethical clothing company Palava. I bought tweed trousers from Brora and jumpers from Hades with band slogans across them, a pretty lilac cardigan from Zara, vintage jeans from Levis and two black taffeta skirts from H&M's collaboration with Beirut-based designer Sandra Mansour. I found shirts by Ines de la Fressange for Uniqlo, a gorgeous grey fake fur coat at Hush and a beautiful black lace dress from Self-Portrait, and added all to my basket. I bought turbans and headwraps in every colour and hue from gold to black, not for-getting all the possible patterns in-between.

Best of all, I became Margaret Howell Woman in reality, buying a smart pair of trousers, a navy cable knit and two shirts. I might not move from Perivale to the imaginary potter's cottage in Corn-wall but I could put on the clothes and pretend I was there while feeling as though one long-held fashion dream had finally come true.

At this point, more than one eyebrow is probably being raised. After all, we're constantly being told about the evils of fast fashion and the importance of ethical shopping. This is not supposed to be the year for self-indulgent shopping or 'emotional' spending sprees but rather a period of reflection where you go through your wardrobe, work out what you actually like to wear and dress accord-ingly. To which I can only reply yes, fair enough, but in the kingdom of cancer different rules apply. There is something about knowing that you are dying which changes the way you respond to things. Obviously I can only speak for myself here, while acknowledging that plenty of other people living with metastatic cancer do not choose to splurge, thinking it a crazy thing to do when you can't guarantee how long you will be around.

My own experience, however, is that I want desperately to spend the last few months of my life looking as good as I can. It doesn't matter to me in the slightest that Covid and the subsequent lockdown means that only Kris, the children and the doctors and nurses treating my disease get to see my different outfits. For, ultimately, I believe that style, the clothes you choose to put on, the things that you fall in love with, have nothing to do with other people. You wear them for yourself. Fashion might be a serious business but wearing it should always be fun.

That simple understanding is the reason that it took stage IV cancer to remind me of how much I loved clothes. For as my world narrows and the end hovers in sight, so I wish to look as good as I can. Like Reality Nirvana Tuttle, I have always embraced my many different fashion personas – I can only hope that I continue to unearth more in the months still to come.

New York
by Brendan Connellan

SARAH EXPLODED INTO MY LIFE LIKE THE COMET THAT SHE WAS AND THE FIRST DAY WAS LIKE ALL THE REST THAT WOULD FOLLOW. She was the sun and the storm all at once and I liked her straight away. The joke was that I was supposed to be protecting her, but I knew better after five minutes.

I hadn't long been in New York when my dad called to tell me that a cousin I had never met was moving to the city. He was very keen that I get her off on the right foot. Yes, London was a big city too but this was the mid-Nineties and he seemed to think there were crack addicts and gun battles whichever way you turned in New York. The place I wanted to take her, he would have given a big, fat 'no' to, so I kept it vague. At the very least, it would tell me something about her and there was always the chance she might like it.

The only way to watch live football in those days was to go to a bar at eight in the morning. It was like stepping through a portal into an alternate universe behind the closed door and the covered windows. It wasn't for the meek. Outside, the pinked and powdered were jogging or walking dogs and planning their mimosas. They could have that. I was more interested in the ones who hadn't seen a bed for two days and were only keeping themselves awake by downing pints, throwing elbows at each other and running in and out of the bathroom for a touch up. Sarah liked it from the first second. She loved it.

The idea was to introduce her around and ease her into it but she didn't need the hand-holding. She was a magnet. Everybody came to her like she was the Duchess of Kent. I had to bow out ten hours later while I could still remember my name but I turned around at the door to check she was safe and saw her bang in the middle of a moshing circle, her head thrown back in laughter, a ciggie in one hand, a vodka tonic in the other and I knew she was going to be alright. It was New York that should be worried.

We saw a lot of each other because Sarah was so full of life; the day and night lost half of its colour when you were away from her so I came back to her like a yo-yo. I'd never met anybody who talked so much and with such conviction. It was a full-contact sport being anywhere near her. I needed to be ready to dodge ash flicked in my face when she got extra excited. And good luck trying to get a word in if she had something she needed to say. It was the time of *Trainspotting* and Chemical Brothers so there was always the thud, thud, thud in the background and the sense that everything was moving very fast and it was wonderful to be young and right in the thick of it. She loved every-thing about the city and said yes to any suggestion. We'd sit in the cheap seats at Yankee Stadium and still be there when the lightweights had bailed, just so we could hear Sinatra sing 'New York' at the end. Then we'd sway together at the pole as the express train hurtled us back downtown, marvelling that all of this was at our beck and call and that we were part of it, we were New Yorkers in the making.

And, boy, did she have opinions. We both devoured books like we needed them to breathe and would take the time to chase down whatever the other recommended, though we did differ at times. The very last thing she said to me was on text and it was to tell me I was wrong and that a book that I had just suggested was good was, in fact, very bad. We did, however, agree that *The Secret History* was the best book ever written. I do remember risking my neck one steaming hot afternoon when I came into my tiny apartment to find her sprawled out on my bed with her head stuck in the pages and her feet mushing up against my pillow. I have a thing about where I put my head so it was a very tough call because it would be like taking a golf club and smacking a lion in the face with it. I regard it as one of the greater achievements of my life that I somehow managed to slide her feet off to the side without her losing her place.

I can't remember why it was that she was going to be staying over one night, just that she needed to meet some friends in a bar first and mumbled that one of them might be coming back with her. I wasn't loving this because it was just one single room with a slanting floor but it was presented to me as a statement rather than a question so I didn't make a big thing of it. I had to be up early so I didn't go with her but I was woken by giggles and belches in the middle of the night and the whiff of a thousand cigarettes. I was able to make out Scottish accents, Russian, maybe some Indian and a few other ones too. I kept my eyes closed but it felt like there were enough to field a hockey team.

When the alarm went off, I eased myself out of bed and tried not to trip over the seven women sprawled on top of each other, somehow squeezed onto the one yoga mat in varying states of undress. It was like a Delacroix painting of a harem in Morocco but without the plump cushions. I had to somehow shower, dress and exit without any of them opening their eyes to see this strange man standing over them and screaming in fright. In the one moment when my back was turned to brush my teeth, two of them sprang up like dolphins and were in my bed and snoring before I'd even rinsed. When I got home, there was no sign of any of them having ever been there. But then, there was always magic and mystery whenever Sarah was involved.

When Sarah came back to New York years later for part two, the remix, she was a few months away from giving birth and had a husband in tow. I had never expected to have her nearby again so this was good news on multiple fronts and gave me an excellent reason to camp out in Brooklyn. It wasn't long after Ruby was born that we all went to the Monmouth Park race track and what an experience it was: a smiling and becalmed new-born, the pounding of hooves and the ringing of the register when the picks came in.

Perhaps it was that glimpse of tranquillity that lulled me into thinking it would be smooth sailing when they dropped Ruby off for me to mind as they headed to a viewing of the BAFTAs. Though I should have been suspicious that they moved so fast in the hand-off, leaving me with just a vague recommendation to sling a bit of bottle at her if she started to wail. All of a sudden, I was left with this wary infant eyeing me thoughtfully, assessing my parental skills. I didn't score well. I don't think any child has every cried louder or longer and it started from the moment that the taxi pulled away.

It was bad. Neighbours were banging on my wall. I needed to get her out of there before the cops broke down the door. I barrelled through the foyer pushing the pram like I'd just robbed a shopping trolley and the concierge gave me that disappointed look you give something after one benefit of the doubt too many. I did loops around the park next door and even the guys sleeping off their hangover there looked up from the ground to shake their heads at me. Ruby didn't stop shrieking until five minutes before her triumphant parents returned in their party frocks, all buzzed up and blissful. Sarah was highly amused when I told her. It capped off her evening.

I know that I'm not the only one to be missing Sarah. We all have our own little stories because she was a person who gave without measuring out the portions. She painted in indelible ink so the memories of her come back fresh and vivid and it still feels like she might walk in the door. To borrow from Whitman, she 'contained multitudes' and she made our lives richer just by passing through them. Some people live longer but not so well, not so fully, and it was a grace to all of us that she let us share her for the time we were given. I hope she knew how much she was loved. It would have surprised absolutely nobody that she was such a fine sport to the very end, the boxer who just wouldn't stay down and the winner of all that mattered. Till we meet again then, Sarah, keep a seat warm for me and I can't wait to hear all your stories.

The Shadow
Children

IT WAS BITTERLY COLD IN NEW YORK THE DAY THAT MY DAUGHTER IRIS DIED. I had just returned from Los Angeles, where I had been carrying out interviews for the first series of *Game of Thrones*, and Iris had kicked and wriggled throughout. I was 35 weeks into my pregnancy and at the stage when I went to my obstetrician every week for a check-up.

I trudged through the cold filled with happiness – my sister had bought Iris a chestnut red cuddly horse to be called Denman, after the Cheltenham 2008 Gold Cup winner (my eldest, Ruby, had a black one named Dun Doire after another

Cheltenham winner while my son Oisín had a sandy one called Dessie after the great Desert Orchid, winner of the 1989 Gold Cup and four-time winner of the Kempton King George V1 Chase).

Five minutes later, I was throwing up in a bin after my obstetrician gently broke the news that my baby was dead.

It was at that moment, at the age of 38, that I became an adult. Until then, my husband and I had led a breezy sort of life, taking nothing terribly seriously. We moved to New York, had two children in swift succession and raised them in a loving if chaotic household where nothing was so bad it couldn't be laughed off with a shrug, a bad joke or a fatalistic, 'Oh well, it'll work out next time.' Then I held my dead daughter in my arms and there were no jokes to be made.

Many weeks after her C-section delivery, long after I had held her and wept, and clutched the memorial box the hospital made for her with her footprints and her bloodstained blanket and the tiny hat, and wept more, I sat in my doctor's office and heard there was nothing wrong with Iris. No complications, no genetic issues, no explanation for why her heart simply stopped beating.

In some ways, it seemed fitting that she had died during a particularly cold New York January and I took a grim satisfaction in how the bleakness mirrored my mood. It seemed only reasonable that the trees should be bare, the streets part-frozen and the skies a dull grey. I was secretly pleased that New York appeared to be grieving along with me; that the city seemed as frozen as I felt.

Yet it's hard to grieve when you have small children. My three-year-old daughter would strike up conversations with people on the subway: 'My mummy's sad because our sister died,' was a particular favourite. Or: 'I had a sister but she died in Mummy's tummy.' Complete strangers would whisper: 'Oh, I'm so sorry,' reach out for the briefest of gestures and then continue on their way.

My son, at 18 months, was oblivious to what was going on. He expected everything to be as it always was and so I forced myself to horse around, to take him to the playground and chase him, to read stories while he sat on my knee.

Trips around the neighbourhood were fraught. Standing in playgrounds, I would bump into people who had last seen me heavily pregnant: 'Oh, did the baby come already?' they would start to say, before breaking off.

At my daughter's nursery school, one of the other mothers had been due around the same time. By coincidence her baby came a week early, on the day Iris should have been born. I found myself unable to talk to a woman who only a few weeks earlier I had had breakfast with once a week. Her daughter was beautiful. I couldn't stand to look at her face.

Worse was the news that a close friend was unexpectedly pregnant with her third child. As the months ticked by, during this period when the grief was supposed to lessen, I would only have to see my friend for my heart to feel shattered once more.

'The grief of a stillbirth is unlike any other form of grief,' Dr Richard Horton, editor-in-chief of *The Lancet*, wrote early last year. Grief is hardly a competition but Horton is right: stillborn grief is different. It's different because there are no happy memories to sustain you, no sense of who that person was and what they meant to you. Instead, you're left grasping at something permanently just out of reach, that might have been, that should have been, that wasn't.

And no one tells you how to deal with that grief. They don't tell you how to react when you find yourself sitting on a floral chair in a dimly lit room in an avuncular funeral director's office discussing why, even though he is waiving his fee, it will cost almost $1,000 for New York State to cremate your baby. Or what to do when letters start arriving from well-meaning social service groups inviting you to talk to grief counsellors about Sudden Infant Death Syndrome and it becomes clear they've mixed up your dead baby with another child.

Then there was the difficulty tracking down her baptism certificate: under New York State law a stillborn birth does not have to be registered, but I needed some sort of recognition that my beautiful daughter had existed. I couldn't bear the idea that she should leave no impression on this world. And so the Catholic priest at the hospital had baptised her and said we could pick up her certificate from his church. Unfortunately, in the turmoil following her birth, he forgot to tell us which church that might be. For months, my husband Kris phoned different churches in downtown Manhattan, trekking out to each one; at one point, we were given the wrong certificate. Sitting at home, I cracked a wan smile: 'This would appear to be becoming a theme.'

According to the stillbirth charity Sands, 17 babies are stillborn or die shortly after birth every day in the UK; one in four stillbirths remains unexplained. In the US, the National Statistics Office reports that one in every 116 pregnancies ends in a stillbirth, roughly 26,000 still-births each year. Yet stillbirth remains one of the great unmentionable subjects, until it hap-pens to you. Before Iris, I knew only one person whose baby had died in the womb. Afterwards, I knew dozens.

The man in the local deli told my husband how

sorry he was and added that his wife had lost a child in the same way; the receptionist at my GP's surgery said it had happened to her. My obstetrician, who had been such a calming, steady presence throughout the silent delivery, almost broke down the next day when talking of how his own child had been stillborn.

Almost two months after Iris's death, I met a woman I knew vaguely outside my flat. 'Has the baby come already?' she said, a smile spreading across her face. 'No, she died,' I blurted, unable to couch it in less brutal terms. We stood in silence. 'I'm so sorry,' she said, and then, grasping for words of comfort: 'You know, they say when that happens it's probably meant to be.' Unable to speak, I nodded and fumbled my way inside. In the hallway, I screamed.

Because a lot of the time I didn't feel sad or depressed or disconnected; I felt really, really angry. Angry with people who were pregnant, angry with people who had three children, angry with people whose babies hadn't been stillborn, angry with people who tried to empathise by talking to me about their miscarriages, angry even with those who were just trying to help.

With family and friends I was closed in, unable to talk, desperate for them to change the subject and move on. 'How do you feel?' they would ask and I would think: 'Awful, as though my soul has been ripped out of my body – is that what you want me to say?' Instead, I would mutter: 'Oh, OK, not great, but you know . . .' and hope that they would leave me alone. I didn't want to share my experiences, to talk about how I felt, to discuss grief. I wanted to shout until my throat was raw and weep until my eyes swelled shut. I wanted to hit things and people. I began to wonder if taking a boxing class would help.

All day, I would sit at my desk trying to write upbeat entertainment articles. And each night, once my children had gone to bed, I would weep uncontrollably over my husband. I had no idea how to talk to Kris. He was so busy keeping it all together, because one of us had to. Going to work, putting the kids to bed, preparing dinner and then holding me while I wept. 'I just want Iris,' I would say. 'I know, darling, I know.' I wanted to ask him how he felt but every time I formed the words my throat felt blocked. 'Are you OK?' I would whisper in bed at night, knowing he would say 'Yes' even if it wasn't actually true.

Like my daughter, I found myself telling complete strangers what had happened. Sitting with my son at his swimming class, I silenced a changing room by announcing that my third child had been stillborn. Even as I said it, I knew it was at best self-indulgent and at worst slightly unhinged. But I couldn't stop myself. I was that crazy lady, the one you'd cross the street to avoid, oversharing to such a level that even New Yorkers looked scared.

As the days crept on, I increasingly felt as though I needed to control my grief, to contain it in some way. I was tired of weeping every evening. Tired of standing in the street with tears pouring down my face, unable to speak to well-meaning passers-by. I was tired, too, of the niggling feeling that maybe I wouldn't have coped with three children. Depressed, angry and shouting at my two living children, the creeping thought would worm its way into my head: 'This is why Iris died – because you can't cope with two and you shouldn't have decided to have a third.'

'There are books that can help you,' my obstetrician had said that first awful morning when I woke in the hospital, my thoughts reduced to the phrase: 'My daughter is dead.' He wrote down a list. I glanced at the titles: *When Bad Things Happen to Good People*, *Coping After Miscarriage and Stillbirth*.

For most of my life, books had provided the answer to all my problems. I had comfort novels for when I felt sick, fast-paced crime stories for those moments I didn't want to think, old favourites I turned to repeatedly through broken hearts and work disappointments, read and reread in good times and bad. But now I didn't know where to start. Comfort reads failed to comfort; new novels were put down one or two pages in; nonfiction seemed too real and fiction too unreal.

I walked in a daze to Barnes & Noble and sat on the floor surrounded by a pile of books pulled at random from the self-help shelves. Books about grief and loss, books about healing and moving on, books specific to stillbirth. I flicked through the pages hoping for a jolt of recognition, a sense that the author understood how I felt. None of them worked. I turned to literary examinations of grief: Joan Didion and C. S. Lewis and Joyce Carol Oates. Yet these books, though often beautifully written, left me equally cold. This was *their* experience of grief, movingly rendered, but ultimately without meaning to me.

For the first time in my life books were failing me. I found myself unable to look away from newspaper reports of celebrities who had lost their children in the same way, reading endless articles on Amanda's loss and Lily's heartbreak. Yet even these similar sad stories, while filling me with a ghoulish sense of companionship, seemed removed.

I went to church, grasping at the Catholic faith of my childhood. The first day we walked in, leaving my two children with their grandmother, they were having a mass baptism. I left hurriedly, rushing for the door. My increasingly concerned husband suggested counselling. I sat at home day after day and willed myself to pick up the phone, but I never made the call. The thought of sitting in a room with strangers and discussing Iris made my skin itch.

Finally, and in desperation, I began to look on the internet. In the early days following Iris's death, Kris had spent some time looking through sites dealing with stillbirth loss but I've never felt that comfortable online. I have no Facebook account, I'm not great at social media and I'd always believed if something truly dreadful happened I would have my family and friends. My mother, sister and brother travelled to New York in the aftermath of Iris's death. My father wrote me a letter so beautifully worded it made me weep. My closest friends crossed the Atlantic, taking precious time out of busy lives to sit with me. In return, I barely spoke.

For all their compassion, I craved the anonymity of strangers. I spoke a couple of times on email to Jess, who had talked about her experience of stillbirth on a friend's website. Her daughter was also called Iris and I started reading her blog, 'After Iris'. Sparse, angry, often extremely funny, it made me weep, yes, but also laugh in recognition. From there, I tracked down more sites and found myself increasingly in contact with other people whose babies had died.

Alice, author of the blog 'Stillborn, Still Standing', put me in touch with Rachel, who, like me, had had two young children before losing her third. Another friend passed on the phone number for a woman whose first child had been stillborn. A woman I knew in passing stopped me in a coffee shop and gave me the email of a male friend who had set up a stillbirth support group after the death of his child. Jess directed me to Glow in the Woods, the site for 'babylost parents' she contributed to, and also to her friend Angie's beautiful, brutal blog 'Still Life with Circles', which runs the Right Where I Am project, in which parents discuss the stage of grief they are at.

And suddenly the world seemed a little less frozen. It wasn't as difficult as going to a therapy group but the result was the same. There were people I could talk to. When Rachel first phoned me, we talked for more than an hour, veering between laughter and anger as we discussed every last detail of our dead daughters.

My online acquaintances were generous with both time and advice. No question seemed too small or outburst too big. They had all been there; they understood how difficult it was to get through the day without crying, how great the struggle between pulling myself together and letting it all fly apart.

For the next couple of months I emailed Rachel and Jess back and forth. Some of those emails were emotional outbursts. 'I was thinking of you this morning – I don't know why, but the lovely weather is somehow making me feel even more sad,' I wrote to Rachel in early June. Others were practical. 'I can't decide whether or not to have a ceremony for Iris, what did you do?' I asked both of them on separate occasions. 'Did you go to a support group?' 'What do you think of counselling?' 'Does this pain lessen?' 'Do I even want it to go away?'

'It feels really odd to me that whole days go by where I barely think of Iris and then I get this wave of extreme emotion and find myself howling hysterically,' I emailed Jess in March. Her response made me feel that I might be able to cope with the pain. 'It doesn't ever go away,' she wrote, 'but it did change for me. It shifted away from the hideous rawness I felt in the early weeks.' I had the sense of some small but hopeful shoot pushing its way slowly through the concrete weight of my grief.

I still wanted Iris. I still dreamed about her, tried to picture her, imagined what she would have been like, but I no longer felt as though I was encased in sorrow. I still looked at the memorial box but I no longer needed to obsessively go through it. Then we travelled back to the UK for a holiday and, in addition to seeing family and friends, Kris and I were able to spend some time alone. We talked about Iris then, but we also talked about silly things and found ourselves beginning to laugh. For the first time in months, I started to imagine a return to normality, to those chaotic family afternoons, to weeping with laughter and not loss.

Throughout it all, I still knew that there was a community of people who understood what I was going through. I talked to them less as my grief became less overwhelming, but it helped to know that they were always just an email away.

Jess was right when she told me that the pain would change. It has, and with the change has come holidays and laughter and the bad jokes of old. Yet throughout it all, Iris is still present and I will not wish her away. For the 35 weeks that I carried my second daughter inside me I was gloriously, life-burstingly happy. I cannot change her story but I carry her with me still.

I carry her dead brother Rory as well. For, after our return to the UK in 2012, Kris and I decided to try again. I had always found it easy to conceive during our marriage and in no time I was pregnant. Then, 20 weeks into my pregnancy, I went to the lavatory and started to bleed huge clots. I realised I was miscarrying and called my sister (Kris was at work and would take too long to get there). She drove me to Charing Cross Hospital, where they began the induction. Kris arrived and I held my perfectly formed but dead son for half an hour and, as with Iris, sung him on his way.

Foolishly, I had thought that the pain and the grief would be far less than with Iris. In reality, it was in some ways much worse. For starters, he was so small that I couldn't cremate him by himself but instead we had to attend a mixed ceremony cremation at Golders Green Crematorium filled with other grief-stricken couples. The ashes were mixed together so could not be taken home. There was, however, some consolation in that Rory was scattered over the Golders Green Garden of Remembrance, joining illustrious stars from rabble-rousing author Kingsley Amis and the groundbreaking founder of psychoanalysis Sigmund Freud to Sid James, the cackling star of the Carry On film series, and the great Irish playwright Séan O'Casey, author of *Juno and the Paycock* and *The Plough and the Stars*. The hospital also gave me a small amount of personal things – a hat, a blanket and footprints – which I added to Iris's box, feeling that they should be together.

That Christmas, my sister made us two beautiful decorations with Iris and Rory's names on them to hang on the Christmas tree. We have hung them every year since, the last decorations before the star at the top, and I hope that Kris and the children will continue that tradition when I am gone.

Over time, I began to think of Iris and Rory as the shadow children. It wasn't a depressing concept. Instead, I saw them running ahead of Ruby and Oisín. They were the playful shadows running in front, calling them out to play. It was a comforting idea and one that gave me succour whenever I felt a shudder of grief. As their mum, I will always carry them with me, just as I will carry Ruby and Oisín, until the day I can lift them no more.

Manchester, So Much To Answer For
by Alexa Baracaia

SARAH WAS INITIALLY JUST A NAME SCRIBBLED ON A
SCRAP OF PAPER THAT I HAD WHEN I LANDED – MID-TWEN-
TIES, ALONE, MILDLY PANICKY – IN MANCHESTER.

I had jumped ship from my first journalism job
in London (and from a faltering relationship) to
join the gossip diary at the *Manchester Evening
News*. Sarah was already working as a features
writer at the paper and had been prepped about
my arrival by a mutual acquaintance, although
we'd never met.

A fellow Londoner in exile, she greeted me with
cocktails and friendship. On my first night in town,

she told me to meet her at the Restaurant Bar & Grill on John Dalton Street. It was then a new and thrillingly lofty marble, glass and mirrors hangout that became a regular haunt over the months that followed, being a handy skip over the road from the *MEN* offices.

I remember a vast table, my glass being filled before I had even taken my seat. I can still hear the thrum and clatter of the place and summon that not unpleasant chlorinated smell you get from indoor water features. I remember, too, copious bottles of prosecco (maybe champagne? We were stupidly profligate with money we didn't have) and instantly and raucously bonding over laughter and cigarettes. Manchester was going to be OK.

I've been trying to give form to one quintessential memory of Sarah. Enduring are blurry 4ams drinking whisky (it 'had' to be Laphroaig), listening to Gram Parsons and Etta James among the detritus of her Salford flat – books, CDs, fags, Christ only knows what else – on a weekday work night. When she got married, I gathered photos of us strewn amid the chaos for a hen weekend gift organised by her closest friends, mocking them up as a magazine cover with the title 'Hell Decoration'. The state of that flat was legendary.

More than once we crawled to our beds at 5am before heaving ourselves out again for bleary 7am starts. How did we even do that?

Evenings would begin with refinement over cocktails at the Bar & Grill, in the chequered lobby of the Midland Hotel or at the Lowry, and end watching *Corrie* stars bawl out karaoke in the gloriously light entertainment surrounds of the Press Club after hours.

Sarah would like nights out to wind up in her living room, where she could sit barefoot, shoes cast to opposing corners, tumbler of drink at her heels, ciggie in one hand, rifling with the other through the teetering piles of CDs to find the next tune that told some wonderfully tragic tale of southern states woe, heartbreak, death and deliciously sleazy romance – poor Billie Joe plummeting from the Tallahatchie Bridge, the tragically jilted groom of a thousand-dollar wedding, Lucinda Williams's drawling pleas to a game-playing lover.

And there, of course, was Sarah, talking at a pace only she and racing pundits at the final furlong could muster about all the things she was ridiculously, unsurpassably passionate, opinionated and wise about – music, books, religion, food, sport, film, fashion. I've rarely met anyone so spirited and knowledgeable about so much.

Not all nights were like that, although those are the ones that stick. Sometimes we curled on my sofa and soaked up the uproarious drama of *Corrie*'s Gail Platt and her 'Norman Bates with a briefcase', the murderous Richard Hillman. Sarah's taste in TV was equal to her adoration of books: highbrow and lowbrow didn't figure, or they didn't matter, anyway.

We worked and played like only twentysomethings unbound by serious stuff can. Those years are often milestone ones, or turning points at least, and Sarah will forever be a defining person in my life. She was my good and loyal friend through a crappy break-up, and again when I got together with my husband, Paul, joining us on some of our earliest nights out and gossiping approvingly with me over coffee the next day at work.

It was a fine and heady time to be in Manchester. The city was emerging phoenix-like from the devastation of the 1996 IRA bombing; it played host both to the Commonwealth Games and the European Champions League final in the space of two exhilarating years. On football: a die-hard Spurs fan, Sarah also had a soft spot for my own national team, Italy, and would usually place a cheeky bet on them winning whichever international tournament was in the offing. I always appreciated having an ally . . . and it paid off for Sarah, too.

On Friday nights, we would get the train home together from Manchester Piccadilly to Euston, upgrading ourselves to first class to make the most of the 'free' warm gin and tonic. When her parents visited, she invited me and our friend Neil out to a pub lunch. Back in London, she'd ask me along to friends' house parties – sometimes forgetting to mention this key fact to her friends, who, despite this, gamely waved me in with an affectionate eye-roll (typical Sarah).

Some people keep their friendship groups distinct and separate, worrying that they may not get on, or jealously hoarding close pals. Sarah was liberal and free with her friendships and would throw us all into the stockpot of a pub night out or summer barbecue, happy to see everyone mix in.

She had a fiercely fabulous roster of friends who had been by her side for years, since way before I met her, and that's testament to the person that she was. Once you'd found her friendship, you were in it for life. If only life had been that bit longer.

After Sarah died, Kris sent me some of her finished chapters to read. She had told me about her ideas for an essay on how cancer had revived her love of fashion. I had a jolt when I read my name: she talks about feeling like a fish out of fashion water in Manchester.

I'm sorry she didn't tell me then a little more about how she felt. I remember very well the night she references – we looked around and twigged that every other woman in the bar was sporting some variation of floppy cropped cargo pants and heels. It was the early Noughties Manchester uniform; a sort of dollied-up take on the less glossy London All Saints style.

The thing is, Sarah never seemed outwardly insecure about her clothes, even though she often spoke with a certain wistfulness about the outfits she used to wear. I always thought of her as stylish. You would never have described Sarah as polished but she always carried everything off with panache. She rocked a mean shoe.

I wish I had told her that then. Funny that one of my memories from Manchester is of feeling too insecure to go to a party because I thought I'd put on weight and looked shit in my dress. Sarah put me right. We went together, got drunk and laughed at all the half-mast trousers.

 ❧

By the time I joined the *MEN*, Sarah was already building a formidable reputation as a writer. Our features editor at the time, Maggie Henfield, was super-supportive of the young women who worked for her and Sarah was given a wide and diverse brief.

Her repertoire mirrored the giddy range and scope of her interests – she won two Feature Writer of the Year awards on the back of a profile with Primrose Shipman, wife of mass murderer Harold Shipman; a piece on a drugs programme in Strangeways prison and an interview with Bob Monkhouse.

She would charm interviewees with her warmth and enthusiasm for almost any topic under the sun: I have vague memories of her getting on uproariously with James McAvoy on a train and chin-wagging with Carl Barat about his wayward co-frontman's habits at some awards after-party or other.

While Sarah wasn't what you'd describe as ambitious in the conventional way – she wasn't particularly interested in climbing the newspaper hierarchy – she was immensely driven and passionate about her work, and, it goes without saying, hugely talented. It was what she was put here to do and she was exceptionally good at it. As an aside, it's a travesty that she didn't end up in a high-flying staff job. She would have liked that and deserved it.

I do remember Sarah had one very specific goal in her head: to work on a national newspaper by the age of 30.

We both made it back to London just in time – or nearly, anyhow. The facts are a little muddy because it later transpired that Sarah was in fact one year older than me. For some unfathomable reason, she only confessed this when her thirtieth birthday came around and I couldn't understand why she was celebrating 12 months early.

Anyway – she was ensconced at the *Observer* by the start of her thirties and that was quite as it should be.

෴

When I left the *Manchester Evening News*, Sarah commandeered the collection kitty and bought me the most incredible pair of 1950s-style pale pink satin heels. She said she feared to think what gift I might otherwise have got if she hadn't taken over.

She was a force of nature, a true and proper friend, even though time and sometimes oceans and the preoccupations of work and family made meetings far fewer than I would now – knowing this – have wished for.

She was old school: someone who would always pick up the actual phone for a chat or to tell her latest news. Those phone calls now sit sharp as pins on the map of our friendship – I can still picture myself standing on a cig break outside the offices of the *Evening Standard*, where I worked on my return from Manchester, when she rang to tell me she was getting married to Kris (and she couldn't have chosen a better man).

There were other calls to tell me of moves to the States and back again, of pregnancy and birth and loss. She would always phone to tell you the important things in life, never leaving it to chance or to the horror that she perceived Facebook to be (and which she never joined. Twitter was latterly her *métier* and, finally, a short but sweet flurry on Instagram, where she shared ad hoc photos of home, Christmas walks, rose and violet creams, her beautiful kids).

When Sarah rang from New York to ask me to be a godparent to Oisín, she said she knew I wasn't religious but saw it as a way of keeping a close bond with good friends. I was honoured and touched. Her Catholicism was always something that she seemed – to me, at least – to wear lightly: it was deeply important but it wove with ease through the secular threads of her life; or, I should probably say, other people's lives.

I don't know how, but she had reverence for her religion while simultaneously pulling it off with irreverence. I was looking back over old messages, trying to recall events that perhaps I had forgotten, and found her email about Oisín's First Communion: 'Only thing you need to know is that mass is long but you guys can go out if needed & you usually give communion child a card & a tenner (or that's what you do in Ireland).'

She wore furry red Louboutins and a leopard-print stole, I think it was, to her church wedding (followed by a proper party at Dover Street Arts Club). And to think she ever thought she wasn't stylish enough.

Latterly, of course, there was the phone call to say she had been diagnosed with breast cancer and was having a mastectomy. In typical Sarah style, it began with a breezy 'Hey, gorgeous' – oh, how I miss that greeting now – and after a lightning-speed rattle through the fundamentals, she moved on to ask what we were up to and how the kids were. In later calls, she was clearly keen not to linger too long on the intricacies of her illness: 'Oh God, it's so boring, let's talk about other stuff.'

The last time I saw Sarah, Kris, Ruby and Oisín all together was a breezy afternoon in the sunshine up at Ally Pally, ambling around the farmer's market and letting the kids roll about on the grass.

Our last night out was to the theatre, to see Andrew Scott – *Fleabag*'s ultimate sexy priest – in *Present Laughter* at the Old Vic. It was a dazzlingly joyful production, for which I am grateful.

Sarah commandeered the queue for the loo by announcing she had cancer and couldn't possibly hang around waiting. Quite right too. We sat and gossiped through the interval, then hugged good-bye on the platform at Waterloo. I texted to make sure she was home safely.

At her funeral, amid the dappled sun and blue-bells in a peaceful Ealing cemetery, I wore new shoes in her honour – not pale pink satin, but near enough.

I hope, I think, she would have approved.

Game of Thrones, Cancer and Me

THE STRANGEST THING ABOUT GETTING BAD NEWS IS THAT YOUR MIND DOESN'T QUITE ACT IN THE EXPECTED WAYS. When my oncologist told me that my triple negative breast cancer, diagnosed in 2017 when I was 44, had metastasised, spreading to my liver and was now stage IV and incurable, the second thought that popped into my head, after the initial throat-closing 'I don't want to leave Kris and the kids', was what if I never find out how *Game of Thrones* actually ends?

You may laugh – and I did, sitting in that sterile appointment room in front of my concerned oncologist and the lovely nurse I'll forever now

171

think of as my own angel of death. It was such an incongruous thought at such a serious time. Yet it also seemed like a legitimate concern.

For once I'd thought about *Game of Thrones*, then all the other things I might never finish rushed through my mind. The series left incomplete, the music I might never listen to, the plays I'd never watch, the conversations I'd never have about books I'd never get to read. Even the possibility that my football team, Tottenham Hotspur, might actually reward a lifetime of faithful trudging to White Hart Lane and Wembley by winning something (I am nothing if not an optimist at heart).

It feels morbid to be thinking this way – after all, my cancer is currently incurable but not terminal – and yet I can't deny that every time I read about a film that's coming next year or the new book by an author I've loved, my initial response is not to think, 'Oh great, I can't wait for that,' but instead to wonder if I'll still be here when it arrives.

Yet it's important to acknowledge those thoughts, grim though they might seem. We talk a lot about fighting cancer and about surviving it, too. Less often about living with and, eventually, in all probability, dying from it. Since last October, when I learned that the cancer had spread, this has been my reality: a daily grind of living with a chronic illness – blood tests, steroids, chemotherapy every three weeks, scan after scan after scan.

It's true, too, that no one reacts in the same way to getting a stage IV cancer diagnosis. There are those who overhaul their diet, who throw out the red meat, the bars of chocolate, the bags of crisps and dedicate their lives to cooking beautiful meals made of kale and turmeric and blueberries and who feel, and often look, much better for it.

There are those whose first thought is to exercise, who head to the gym and pound the pavements and show, repeatedly and admirably, that their bodies are as strong and fit as they were before.

There are those whose overwhelming urge is simply to get into bed and stay there.

There are people who investigate every possible way of staying alive and people who think: 'Sod it, I'm going to live my life as I always have and see what happens next.'

My response when I learned that the cancer was now incurable fell somewhere between all of those.

I'd like to say that the news was shocking enough that I immediately began planning a health overhaul in order to stay alive as long as possible, but the reality is that I am naturally a pretty lazy person and when I heard my oncologist say that at this point treatment was a marathon rather than a sprint, all I could think was that I was terrible at long-distance running at school but pretty good at pelting for the bus, which didn't exactly bode well.

I am not very good at dealing with attempts to talk about my health, however well meaning. For a time, when people would bring up my bad luck, sighing sympathetically with their heads cocked to the side, I would nod extra sincerely and agree that yes, it was terribly bad luck but on the other hand, I'd been very lucky both in love and on the horses and you can't have everything going your way.

That's not to say I haven't taken my diagnosis seriously. It's more that while I have made some effort to eat more plant-based food, have started walking distances every day and am flirting with everything from swimming to yoga, it was – and is – easier for me to live each day much I as did before.

People tell you that when you get this kind of devastating news, conversations take on an almost burnished intensity, you hug those you love harder, live in the moment, love what is left of your life more. It's true, but what they don't say is that sometimes, despite all the treatments, the hours spent giving blood, taking pills, sitting through chemo, the occasionally bone-shattering tiredness . . . sometimes you forget you even have stage IV cancer at all.

It's in those moments that popular culture rushes in. When I was first diagnosed I turned to Jilly Cooper, rereading first her early romances then all the Rutshire Chronicles, from *Riders* to *Mount!* During chemo, I ploughed through boxsets, from *Peaky Blinders* to *Derry Girls*. Post-mastectomy, I survived on a diet of Dorothy Dunnett's Lymond Chronicles, Donna Tartt's *The Secret History*, Leigh Bardugo's Grishaverse books and Sally Beauman's family house saga *Dark Angel*. When reading proved too difficult, thanks to a combination of morphine and pain, I watched old TV series, such as *Glue*, and newer ones like *Save Me* – one of the best things about a lengthy stay in hospital is the chance to catch up with all those programmes you meant to get round to finishing but never quite managed.

Looming over everything, however, was *Game of Thrones*, George R. R. Martin's epic tale about life, death, murder and politics in the Seven Kingdoms of Westeros. Not simply because, entering its final season, it remains television's one true juggernaut, the biggest, most bombastic show of them all, but because if one piece of popular culture could be said to have dominated my life for the past 15 years it is this one.

Even writing that feels weird. Martin's sprawling creation is not my favourite story, nor do I think that either it or the subsequent HBO adaptation are the greatest pieces of art ever made, much as I love them both. But there are some pieces of popular culture that, by some weird alchemy, can come to dominate your life – and *Game of Thrones* has, both for good and bad, dominated mine.

I first came across the series A Song of Ice and Fire almost two decades ago, in my twenties, when I was doing sub-editing shifts in any office that would take me. It was the sort of grinding, monotonous work where you moved from office to office, week after week, and no one really talked to you because you'd soon be gone. Lonely, I spent every lunchtime in nearby cafés reading *A Game of Thrones*, the first of Martin's books, which I'd picked up initially because of its size. I'd never really been a fantasy reader but this was fantasy with a political bent and, crucially, it was big enough to pass the time. From the first page I was hooked.

Some books can do that, providing the literary equivalent of a shot of adrenaline to the heart and making sure that you turn the pages long into the night and first thing in the morning. I finished *A Game of Thrones* in a gulp, sighing over the fate of the Starks and laughing at Tyrion Lannister's bitter one-liners, and promptly moved onto the second book in the saga, *A Clash of Kings*. I was lucky because the year was 2000 and the third book, *A Storm of Swords*, had just been published. I had no idea how long I would then have to wait for volumes four and five. If I had then I would perhaps have paused before devouring it.

What happened next happened partially because of the time. The early Noughties was an era of message boards, of the discovery that you could find people all over the world who shared your interests and obsessions, and talk to them about even the most obscure points. So it was that while slacking off during another lengthy subbing shift (this one at night) I discovered the Westeros message board, A Forum of Ice and Fire. In an age before social media dominance, it transformed my world, bringing me into contact with people across the world and allowing me to hear their opinions and thoughts on everything from obscure points of Westerosi law to real-life global politics. I spent the night of the 2004 US election talking to *Game of Thrones* fans about what would happen and debated politics with people in Memphis and Mumbai.

I was given recommendations for everything

from books and films to where to eat and drink in cities throughout the world. It seems so minor now, but at that time it felt as though the whole world had come closer and anyone could have a say.

The arrival of the television series in 2011 kicked everything up a notch. I covered the press junket for the first series and was asked by the *Guardian* to write a series of weekly recaps of the show. The request came at a very difficult time in my life – three days after the junket my third child was stillborn – yet it also gave me something to cling on to. Barely capable of work, there was a bleak comfort in losing myself in the power struggles of the Seven Kingdoms, this graphically brutal world where no one could be trusted and where words were the sharpest weapons of all. It might seem like an overstatement but writing those recaps helped restore life to me. I loved arguing with the commenters about what had happened and what might happen next. I relished the pressure of having to get each recap online in such a short space of time, as well as the chance to truly lose myself in a fictional world.

I think about those days a lot right now – it's hard not to, given my health. On bad days, it can seem monstrously unfair to have had two still-births (the second was in 2012) and an incurable cancer diagnosis in eight years. I've found some solace in sitting in church – I grew up Catholic and the faith of my childhood is a useful crutch at difficult times, even if I've never been the most devout of practitioners. It helps, too, in my darker moments, to acknowledge that the treatment I've received has been exemplary, from my pragmatic oncologist Dr Laura Kenny to the funny, honest and, above all, incredibly patient nurses on the oncology ward at Charing Cross Hospital and the many, many people there and at Hammersmith Hospital who have patiently tried to extract blood from my recalcitrant veins.

Despite all the difficult times, I'd be lying if I said that the last decade hasn't been the best of my life. I've been lucky in love, fulfilled in my work, surrounded by friends, laughed more than I ever thought possible at the most ridiculous of things. I can say with absolute honesty that I have had a lovely time and I don't regret any of it, not even those dark and slightly desperate days in my late twenties when I mistook the ability to drink long into the night for personality and saw more charm in a series of older men than they ever genuinely exhibited.

It's true, too, that the less time you think you may have left in this world the more you want to intensely experience it. Over the past months, I have been intensely grateful for walks with my dog, giggling hugs from my children, Ruby, 11, and Oisín, 9, coffee with my parents, trips away with my two siblings and more silly conversations with friends than I can count. For uncontrollable laughter and fantastic sex and, most of all, for all the many times that my husband Kris has raised an eyebrow and told me to get over myself and stop auditioning for a part as a dying swan.

I think a lot, too, about something that the late Andrea Levy, author of *Small Island* and *The Long Song*, apparently said. That when her breast cancer stopped being treatable and became stage IV and incurable, she realised she didn't want to spend what was left of her life in a room writing. She wanted, instead, to live.

I understand that and yet I want both. I want to cling to every moment but I also want to read and watch everything I can. Call it a manifesto for the chronically lazy, perhaps, for those of us who have always liked to spend our time transfixed as all that is great and terrible about human life parades across the screen or page, but if I spend what is left of my time lying on a sofa reading I won't feel that I have missed out.

Best of all, while I might not find out how Martin himself intends to finish his series (there are still two long-awaited books to come), I will almost certainly see the TV series of *Game of Thrones* return for its brutal, no doubt bloody and hopefully rewarding conclusion this month. As for Tottenham Hotspur winning the league in my lifetime, that remains too great a step for even the most benign of gods to arrange.

The Observer Years
by Lisa Bachelor

IT HAPPENED IN APRIL AND AGAIN OVER THE SUMMER THEN FOR A THIRD TIME LAST WEEK. I was discussing with the editor of the *Observer* newspaper who we thought might be the best person to write particular pieces we had in mind. Each time I had to stop myself saying, 'Oh Sarah would be perfect for that.'

Sarah and I first met around 20 years ago while both working for the newspaper. They were slightly blurry days filled with rushed deadlines, hectic socialising and immense headaches brought on by too much gin and, I'm sure Sarah wouldn't mind me saying, on her part, copious amounts of whisky. But it wasn't until 2015, when I moved on to the *Observer*'s news desk, that Sarah and I struck up first a working relationship and then, so much more importantly, a fulfilling friendship.

The whole thing could have started badly. Unbeknown to me at the time, Sarah had gone for the same job as me and inexplicably I had got it. When I did find out, I sent her an apologetic email, saying rather wimpishly that I 'hoped she didn't feel peeved at me'. The reply was instant and utterly Sarah: 'Darling, not at all, if I couldn't get it then I was glad it was you, as much to have someone I'm friends with than a random person.'

From that point, we spent the next five-and-half years talking, sometimes in the office, more often over lunch, about everything from books, films, TV programmes, sport and global politics to the school curriculum. We also discussed our home lives. We found common ground in a similar home set up – both in our forties, husband, two children of similar ages and even a dog each bought around the same time. Husband Kris, Ruby and

Oisín were, without a doubt, between them, the best things that ever happened to her and I loved hearing about their lives.

She was an extraordinary storyteller and was equally at home chatting in a pub to a group of middle-aged blokes about her much-loved team Tottenham Hotspur or her passion for horse racing as she was discussing American politics, 'trashy' novels – which she loved – or fashion. She was incredibly clever, funny, kind and generous with her praise. Every email began 'Hey darling' and ended in multiple kisses. Even when she was a bit cross.

Every idea for the *Observer* was special to Sarah and everything she ever came up with (and there was plenty) was delivered with the most enormous amounts of enthusiasm, urgency and knowledge.

She would tell me about up-and-coming authors I had never heard of, programmes I should know about, films 'we' (meaning the *Observer*; it was always 'we' and not 'I' in her pitches) should be covering. She achieved a feat not always easy for a journalist on the news pages of a broadsheet newspaper, which was to fight for and be granted coverage for popular television shows, films and books on a regular basis.

Sarah was an absolutely tireless worker. Sometimes I would still be peeling my coat off, shaking the rain from my hair or bleary eyed with a coffee in hand when she would bounce over on the dot of 9am, or before, bursting with ideas and energy. If she was working from home she would call me at that same hour with the same exuberance in her voice. She also never seemed to switch off. The emails I'd get often amazed me, some of which I reread before writing this piece and made me chuckle. 'Hey guys, just to let you know I am in Jamaica but also around so just let me know if you have any queries/want things to be rejigged.' Another was, 'Just at Ascot so may not be able to reply to things too quickly but will get back to you.' And, 'I'm by the sea with poor Wi-Fi but I really want to chat about this piece. When are you free?'

Yet, despite being known as a prolific writer, it was the pieces she wrote for the *Observer* from her heart in the later years of her life that captivated a new audience.

Before her stunningly candid and moving accounts about her battle with cancer, she had written about stillbirth and the agonising loss of two babies, Iris in 2011 and then Rory in 2012. She wrote about this first for the *Observer* magazine and then in a news piece I commissioned about stillbirth in 2017. Was she OK writing about her own experience, I asked, or would this be too much? 'I am,' she replied. 'I always get a little emotional in the interviews because everyone usually has the same experience but that's part of it.'

The filed copy was a perfect piece – practical and personal in equal parts.

'I talked about Iris alone in the dark of the night and the early hours of the morning – and I did it online,' she wrote. 'For there is something about the anonymity of an internet forum that allows you to speak more honestly than you perhaps can to those who know you best.'

Then there were the pieces about her journey

with cancer. Her honest and ultimately upbeat accounts drew a new audience, often those who were suffering during the same journey as her and appreciated someone voicing their experience so articulately.

These pieces were particularly difficult for me (and I'm sure many people who knew and loved her) to read because, like the passing of her babies, Sarah rarely talked about her illness. I was not surprised to see this sentence in one of her pieces: 'I am not naturally good at dealing with attempts to talk about my health, however well meaning.'

This first became clear to me in March 2018 when she told me she had a breast cancer. I wobbled and then wavered over the right thing to say and yet she batted off any attempts at consoling her, keen to get back to work. Later, in an email, I asked if she had told some mutual friends of ours. In typical matter-of-fact Sarah style, she replied: 'I haven't but I don't mind you telling them because to be honest, it's a hassle having to have the same conversation constantly.'

Then in the late summer of that year, she had

to deliver the even worse news that the cancer had spread to her liver and was now stage IV and incurable. I was on my local high street when she called; the rain was coming down, the traffic was loud and I couldn't hear what she was saying, so I ducked into a side alley. 'It's spread,' she said, when I could eventually hear her. 'I've got an interview lined up this afternoon but I'm not sure I can do it right now.' Of course she shouldn't do it, I said – but even then she made me insist I would line up someone else to do it. She even suggested the right reporter for the piece, adamant that she didn't want to let the interviewee down.

I was always worried about whether she was pushing herself too hard to work so I would often check that she really was sure she wanted to write. I remember her once saying to me that actually she loved working and that it helped and that she was pretty cheerful most of the time. She even seemed to make laughing at her illness acceptable, which I think she really wanted people to feel able to do. Times like when she said, 'Honestly, it would really annoy me to die during the pandemic as I have a very self-indulgent funeral planned.' And Sarah's verdict when doctors decided the treatment she was on wasn't working and they wanted to try a course of steroids instead? 'Boo, weight gain; yay, possible life extension!'

Despite her diagnosis and the rapid progression of the disease, she fought on doggedly and outlived all her doctor's expectations. She never stopped working and would file from her hospital bed, at one point memorably phoning me about a piece while repeatedly berating the nurse who was at her bedside trying to get her ready for a procedure. 'I'm on the phone to my editor, I just need a minute,' she kept insisting as the nurse gently tried to get her to concentrate on the matter in hand.

During the pandemic, life became particularly hard for Sarah as she had to shield herself from another terrible illness she feared might claim her life. Even so, she managed to be positive. 'But it's fine,' she wrote as we discussed lockdown woes once. 'I've never been more glad to live in the suburbs of west London because Kris can take the kids to play Gaelic football up a hill every day for an hour and there's no one there. Plus I have a garden.'

She wrote about this time in her life in another memorable piece for the *Observer* magazine, this time in November 2020, conveying that same positive attitude. It was aptly headlined 'Find Some Part of Each Day to Relish'.

After her diagnosis and before the pandemic, she made sure to pack plenty into the time she did have left with a series of holidays and adventures with Kris and the children. She messaged, typically joyously, from one of these. 'We're in Penzance, literally on the beach, which the kids can't believe . . . have never been to Cornwall before, it's amazing.'

In all the conversations I had with her nearer the end, she never stopped talking about life and never once mentioned death and she always kept her sense of humour.

I honestly miss her so terribly, of course for her outstanding writing, but, far more than that, for her companionship, her humour and her generous spirit. Sometimes I see a photo of her and it's like I can see her standing by my desk again, laughing at something that tickled her. When I pass the pan-Asian restaurant where we used to go for lunch my heart sometimes skips a beat – I miss our chats, which were usually about life and politics rather than work, over plates of pad Thai. Near the end, I don't think she enjoyed the food and could only eat a little but she never cancelled a lunch date as I think she loved to chat. And so did I.

I will never forget the words she wrote in a piece for the *Observer* three years ago: 'I'd be lying if I said that the last decade hasn't been the best of my life. I've been lucky in love, fulfilled in my work, surrounded by friends, laughed more than I ever thought possible at the most ridiculous of things. I can say with absolute honesty that I have had a lovely time and I don't regret any of it.'

Titled '*Game of Thrones*, Cancer and Me', it was about her journey through the disease that ultimately claimed her life, and how she drew strength from her unwavering passion for popular culture to give her something to hold onto in dark times.

The piece wasn't miserable, although it made

me cry for a long time afterwards; it wasn't angry or filled with sadness, despite the fact that Sarah had every right to write with all of those emotions. Instead, it was bold, practical, reflective, just a little bit cheeky in parts and utterly witty. In short, it was just like Sarah herself.

Food, Confusing Food

AT NIGHT I DREAM OF FOOD. Fresh spanakopita pies, unctuous pork belly, sharp blood orange and beetroot salad, smooth, soothing dals. All of these dishes and more flash through my mind, so close that it feels that I can reach out and taste them. In the morning, I wake up and my mouth feels full of ashes. The food doesn't exist and, even if it did, the cancer plays havoc with my taste and appetite. Sometimes things feel too sweet, other times too salty. There are days when I can devour three-course meals and days when I can only eat an apple. For someone who has always enjoyed their food, even when I was a heavy smoker, it is an experience close to torture.

Nor is it just the food I miss. I love having people over for long, chatty lunches or dinners, yet frustratingly no longer have the energy to organise them, even if we weren't living in lockdown.

Given all this, what's a greedy woman to do? In my case, I have developed an addiction to cookbooks.

I bought cookbooks about Russia, Thailand and Greece. I read my way through Meera Sodha, Sabrina Ghayour and Honey and Co. I bought vegetarian cookbooks and vegan ones too. I read about all aspects of African-American food in Toni Tipton-Martin's *Jubilee*, a particular delight. I discovered Sam Sifton, food editor for the *New York Times*, whose *See You on Sunday* is full of practical, tasty recipes. I fell in love with Rachel Roddy's beautiful writing and Italian recipes and, like every other middle-class lockdown cliché, devoured Nigella's warm and witty *Cook, Eat, Repeat*. Then, when I'd read my way through the new cookbooks, I turned back to my old favourites: Diana Henry, Joanna Weinberg and the ubiquitous but inspiring Ottolenghi.

I travel the world through these books. Imagining the bustle of India and the deep blue calm of the Greek island of Ikaria, whose inhabitants are among the longest-living in the world. I dreamed of the perfect aperitivos followed by genuine Roman *amatriciana* devoured with Kris in one of the tightly packed Testaccio tavernas Roddy so lovingly describes, or eating plate after plate of meze in that grand dame of Europe, Istanbul. My dreams take me to cafés in Paris and tapas bars in Seville. They let me linger over Thai street food, devour borscht in Ukraine and eat fresh langoustines with soda bread in Ireland.

Of course, one of the great things about living in a city like London is that most of these foods are easily available. The problem is that my appetite is not always quite so compliant, which makes dreaming about food easier than actually eating it.

എ

I have always been, if not a greedy person, then one with a healthy appetite and always as interested in the social aspect of eating as much as the food itself. I have never divided food into good and bad or talked of guilty pleasures. Instead, I have eaten what I wanted, when I wanted and not worried about weight or looks. That might seem unlikely but I mention it because I started to care when my cancer spread and I was put on steroids. Photos from this time show a small rotund person with a huge moon face and I can barely bring myself to look at them. It was probably the only time when I didn't want to have people over for dinner and drinks and long evenings laughing into the night (if I'd known that a pandemic was looming, I might have decided differently and thrown my vanity to the side).

My love of entertaining and food dates back to my childhood when I would watch my mum, a microbiologist in the Scottish Borders, preparing formal dinner parties for her colleagues and those of my father, who was professor of surgery at Edinburgh University. It was an era when food was expected to look fancy, with lots of heavy sauces and three courses, the centrepiece an extremely fancy-looking and rich dessert – my mum's speciality involved raspberry mousse topped with raspberries and encircled by sponge biscuits. Watching the preparations, they did often seem more hassle than they were worth and yet there was something magical about the whole affair. The elaborate dinners, the table placement, the chat about everything and nothing.

This feeling that food and parties went hand in hand and were part of life's joys was strengthened by my dad's annual Christmas party, a lively event to which the whole department was invited, where the children all hung out together, stuffing our faces with crisps, sweets and cocktail sausages, watching TV, playing games and generally mucking about, while the adults enjoyed a drink or two elsewhere.

Of course, life wasn't all high entertainment and parties. My mum still had to feed the three of us while working. She did her best, although not everything was a success. Over 30 years later, I can still remember the horror of fried liver and how my sister and I would hide it in our cheeks before sneaking to the loo and spitting it down there.

There were other much nicer meals: expertly cooked Sunday roasts, a pork and mustard dish that became known as 'the meal we always quarrel over' because for some reason we all fell out every time we ate it and wonderful Victoria sponges and summer puddings. For a time when my Granny Tea (so called because of her love of tea) lived with us – she died of pancreatic cancer when I was ten – there were perfect Yorkshire puddings and roast potatoes.

Granny Tea, a.k.a. Alice, was a Lancashire woman who grew up in Bolton and initially worked at one of the mills near there before training to become a nurse and moving to London, where she met my Scottish grandfather, Max. Her granny flat at the back of our house felt like a benign witch's lair in which she made me apple dolls and allowed me to watch *Excalibur* while she drank tea and ironed clothes.

This being the late 1970s and early 1980s, the

cupboards also held plenty of odd and exciting produce: Smash and tubs of Nesquik, Viennetta in the freezer for special occasions and, if we were lucky, even a bit of Angel Delight. What we didn't have was a SodaStream: I was insanely jealous of a primary school friend whose family did. We sat in her garden as her dad brought us bottles of fizzy drinks and it seemed like the perfect life.

Sadly, my mother was never going to buy one due to a latent distrust of all things American. She will vigorously deny this (I can see her shaking her head right now) but as evidence, she repeatedly says that two things she has never done are wear a pair of jeans and drink Coke, both of which are quintessentially American.

Yet she didn't despise modern technology. I can vividly remember the arrival of the micro-wave, seen in our house as a life-changing invention. Suddenly, the house filled up with packets from Marks & Spencer: tagliatelle dishes ready in minutes, trays of vegetables that simply required you to puncture the film several times and then stick them in the blessed machine. Even bacon, previously the preserve of my dad, who did a mean fry up, was placed in it. There were takeaways too, baked potatoes from SpudULike being a regular and oddly exciting Saturday lunch.

Despite this love of food, as a teen I wasn't particularly interested in cooking any. There was a brief attempt to be grown-up with a dinner party for my sixteenth, which I think was based around a horribly rich dish of duck in cherry sauce, but otherwise the most I did during this period was burn toast. That all changed with university. I had to be able to cook for myself – it was either that or live on a diet of cheesy chips, sausage rolls and takeaways (including that infamous Scottish special: the deep-fried pizza). Luckily, in this hour of need, I found a saviour. Nigel Slater's *Real Fast Food* was published in 1992 and showcased a whole new way of cooking. It was here that I learned the basics, from cooking a decent roast chicken to which herbs to use and when.

From there developed an obsession. I learnt basics from *The Good Housekeeping Cookbook*, poured over Delia and devoured *Madhur Jaffrey's*

Indian Cookery, which opened up a new and exciting world. My flatmates and I had countless Sunday lunches, all of which started sedately before descending into typical student chaos, but which were great fun.

Post-university in Berlin and New York, I had little time or space to throw the dinner parties of my dreams but on my return to London I lived with three of my closest friends and there were parties galore, though many of them admittedly without much food involved. More importantly, we cooked for each other, trying things out and perfecting old favourites from beef stroganoff to a particularly tasty sausage casserole.

When Kris and I moved in together there were more lunches and dinners. I discovered Joanna Weinberg's *How to Feed Your Friends with Relish* and joyfully cooked my way through it, providing long lunches that bled into the evening, recalling the meals at St Andrews a decade before. It wasn't until we moved to New York, however, that my love of food and entertaining really took hold.

In Brooklyn, I had a blank canvas. We started

meeting people in the neighbourhood and the natural thing was to invite them over for lunch or dinner. We had people over for everything from Thanksgiving to simple barbecues in our humid, tiny, mosquito-friendly backyard (the latter was not as unpleasant as I've made it sound, you just had to be well prepared with candles, bug spray and the Elizabeth Arden oil that New Yorkers swore kept the beasts away). There were laughter-fuelled Christmas meals – including a memorable one where our close friend Rik and my dad attempted to make custard with no success – and a particularly raucous Easter lunch which went on far too long but also provided a ton of juicy gossip. There were long, leisurely evenings with my Irish-American cousins and quiet, intimate evenings where Kris and I talked long into the night.

This being New York, we also ate out, enjoying the many different brunches on offer in Cobble Hill, Fort Greene, Red Hook and Park Slope. But it is the home meals that linger longest in my mind, as I realised that the simple act of enjoying a meal could and did go on to form the building blocks of deep friendships that endure to this day, regardless of the ocean between us.

It helped too that we lived near Atlantic Avenue, with its bustling array of Middle Eastern shops, the star of which was Sahadi's, with its trays of juicy olives, tangy anchovies and salty blocks of fresh feta cheese. There were other delights too – a wonderful fishmonger which made addictive fishcakes, a family-run butchers where almost anything could be ordered and two great farmers' markets, one at Grand Army Plaza and the other in Fort Greene. Over time, it became a habit to stroll down to these with the children, browsing the stalls before stopping for brunch on the way home. These days, when farmers' markets are everywhere and the talk is all about sustainability and fresh, local produce, such activity seems mundane but in 2008 there was a marked contrast between Brooklyn and Manhattan, with the former far more to the forefront of the change in eating patterns. It is also true that this was a very middle-class way of eating and we didn't always stick to it, often resorting to quick dishes of tins of beans purchased from Key Food and supplemented with salad and cheap vegetables.

What I really took from my time in New York, however, wasn't a lesson in how to eat but rather the notion of food as a shorthand for camaraderie. I loved that sharing a good bottle of wine and eating something prepared with thought and love could bring people together and even create new bonds. For me, the kitchen was the bustling hub of the house. Our ground floor happened to be open plan, which helped, but even if it wasn't, I still firmly believe that there is little more enjoyable than sitting around a worn kitchen table and chatting with family and friends.

While I had had very few side effects with my initial chemotherapy that all changed once the cancer spread. I developed mouth ulcers, found my appetite fluctuating and went through periods where nothing tasted right. I am so thankful that these times have been interspersed with moments when I could devour delicious three-course meals – one of the few good things about the pandemic lockdown being the restaurant meal kit. But when eating was all but impossible, reading recipes and imagining how they might turn out was a lovely respite.

On my better days I cooked from them too. Simple but beautifully flavoured chicken recipes from Diana Henry, fragrant vegetarian meals by Anna Jones for my daughter, Cypriot comfort food from Georgina Hayden's lovely second book, *Taverna*. In the run-up to Christmas, I cooked my way through Nigella's *Cook, Eat, Repeat*, making everything from oxtail stew to the rightly celebrated fish finger bhorta. Early on in lockdown, Kris and I had decided that, while expensive, a Big Green Egg – a ceramic charcoal grill and smoker – would be a worthwhile investment, and so it proved. We fell into a comfortable rhythm where he cooked the meat and fish and I dealt with the sides and Ruby's meal, a situation that reminded me once again that one of the great pleasures of life is the sense of a shared experience and cooking together can be one of the most enjoyable experiences of all.

These memories sustained me when the cancer worsened, making it increasingly difficult for me to help. A series of infections led to prolonged stays in hospital where I would dream about food while trying to eat the monotonous meals served in the ward. It was during these stays that I developed my out-of-control meal-kit habit. Lying alone in bed at night I'd think, 'Oh, I really fancy a Middle Eastern spread or an Indian curry,' and with one click I could order them to be at the house when I returned. We ate meals from Galvin and Petersham Nurseries, thanks to online service Restokit, and my children thrilled to the retro pleasures of the cheese fondue thanks to The Cheese Bar. Throughout it all, I still dreamed of food and wished that I could cook from my many books rather than simply reading them and salivating over what was within.

But reading them did still provide succour. I could still travel to different countries in my head, still imagine what meals would taste like and still dream about cooking from those books once again. In the meantime, Kris proved a willing accomplice, trying new things and, helped by my goddaughter Sefi (with who we had formed a bubble), dealing with various meal kits at the weekend.

Luckily, while my appetite fluctuated, I've never entirely lost it and was always able to eat at least one largish meal each day. This became increasingly important as I began to get regular infections resulting in prolonged periods in hospital. Finding the food increasingly inedible, I relied on Kris for my evening meal, which could be anything from Italian to Indian and was always delicious.

I came out of hospital clear about what I wanted to do next. My priority would be to teach my children the basics of cooking so that the burden didn't entirely fall on Kris once I had gone. There are, after all, only so many meal kits a person can make. That's not to say that he relied entirely on them – in fact, he is a very good cook who can make anything from a superlative shepherd's pie to a lovely seafood sizzle of clams, mussels and occasionally langoustines. It couldn't hurt to have some help, however, especially from Ruby, as a vegetarian. To be fair, at 13, she already made tasty chickpea traybakes, noodle bowls and a great pasta with tomato sauce and feta, which her brother adored and regularly requested. I wanted her to expand her repertoire – luckily, she is someone who genuinely likes both vegetables and the kick of umami. I needed her to learn how to make a béchamel sauce and cauliflower cheese, to make carrots and parsnips interesting and to experiment with leeks, Jerusalem artichokes and celeriac. I would teach her how to make curries, soup and comforting stews, to widen her cooking beyond chickpeas towards lentils, split peas and the cannellini bean cakes she loves.

Oisín is even easier. He's not an adventurous eater but he is very keen to help out and learn how to cook. I would teach him how to roast a chicken and then use the leftovers for stock; how to make the sausages and mash he so loves and how to cook Nigella's ham in coca cola, probably his favourite meal of all. His dad would teach him how to make steak and chips, spaghetti bolognese and shepherd's pie, in addition to showing him how to cook on the Green Egg. Finally, I would give both children my Nigel Slater, Diana Henry and Claire Thomson cookbooks and let Ruby pick her favourite vegetarian books.

This, then, is my plan, a celebration of the food I have most enjoyed and a way of passing my love down the line. For me, food has always been a way of celebrating. In my darkest moments it has sustained me. For even when I couldn't eat, I could always read about it and imagine that I was sitting in an Italian taverna or eating street snacks in Mumbai. Those dreams got me through some of the darkest periods of my disease and it is for that reason that I raise a non-alcoholic glass to toast food, wonderful, celebratory food.

Cancer During Covid

NOVEMBER 2020

THE STRANGEST THING ABOUT HAVING AN INCURABLE ILLNESS DURING A TIME OF PANDEMIC IS THE WEIRD BUT UNAVOIDABLE SENSE THAT EVERYONE HAS FINALLY CAUGHT UP WITH YOU. As people started talking about how worried they were, how they couldn't stop thinking about the virus, how difficult life now seemed, how isolated, the temptation to say, 'Hey guys, welcome to my world!' was overwhelming.

This had never felt more pertinent than last month, when social media lit up with Breast Cancer Awareness memes and pink ribbons and talk of fighting and beating the disease. For those of us with stage IV cancer, such messages seem beamed in from another planet. As the campaign group MetUpUK points out, 31 people die every day from metastatic breast cancer and countless more of us live each day with a disease that has a median survival rate of two to three years – a rate that drops considerably if you have a cancer that began as a triple negative breast cancer, as mine did. Yet our stories, which might force people to face the uncomfortable truth that we are not 'winning' the 'fight', are rarely told.

The thing about living with stage IV cancer is that it's ever present. You can be doing the most mundane of tasks – cooking dinner, chatting to your children or lying on the sofa reading a great book – and suddenly the unwelcome thought will pop into your mind: 'Oh, I have an incurable disease and one day it's going to kill me.' These thoughts are at their strongest during situations such as the last lockdown and, now, the current one.

When the first lockdown was introduced I read the government's guidelines and looked at their ratings chart of vulnerable people, only to discover that because I had an incurable cancer and was being treated with intravenous chemotherapy I was rated a nine – the most vulnerable category.

This seemed monumentally unfair. I had a job. I walked my dog. I met my children after school and cooked dinner and occasionally even managed to overcome my tendencies towards antisocial behaviour by actually going out and seeing people for coffee and dinner and drinks. Yet according to the guidelines, I was more at risk than people who needed a full-time carer or had an underlying condition that made them particularly vulnerable to Covid. And because of that I was supposed to isolate myself from my family, to spend my time in the bedroom attic having my food dropped outside and occasionally opening a window to ensure a breath of fresh air.

Much as I have long entertained fantasies of becoming Miss Havisham and sitting in a rocking chair declaring doom to all who visit, these measures seemed something of a step too far. For a start, they coincided with my cancer failing to respond to the oral chemo that had kept it under control for the previous few months, which meant I would have to leave the house if only to get my intravenous chemo treatment. In addition to this, an unpleasant new development meant that I would also require regular hospital visits to treat ascites, a build-up of fluid in my stomach that can occur in patients with advanced liver cancer.

So I formed my own plan. For much of lockdown, I did stay in the house, unless I had hospital treatment, but I also hung out with my family, sat in the garden, continued to work and occasionally, on the advice of my oncologist, took the dog for a short walk on the hill where we live. This time round, when the government advice is less stringent, I shall continue to be cautious while trying to fit in some exercise and live a semblance of normality.

I am lucky in more ways than one. Lucky that my home is way out in west London's suburban zone 4, which means that we have a decent garden and plenty of open space nearby. Lucky that the cancer is in my liver, which has largely allowed me to continue to lead a relatively normal, mostly pain-free life and, most of all, lucky that I continue to receive treatment during this time.

One of the biggest non-Covid issues to arise during the pandemic has been the way in which it has affected cancer patients. People have had their treatment paused or, in some cases, frightened of contracting the virus, chosen to pause it themselves. Procedures have been delayed and even halted. People have ignored lumps or other warning signs, more terrified of Covid than of cancer. There are reports of primary cancers spreading because they weren't caught in time and secondary cancers progressing at a faster rate because the treatment wasn't available to keep the disease in check.

In May, Steven McIntosh, policy director for the leading cancer charity Macmillan Cancer Support, told the *Guardian* that there had been 'a very worrying drop in the number of people coming forward with suspected cancer symptoms to be referred for diagnosis by their GPs', adding that 'as many as 1,900 cases of cancer a week are currently going undiagnosed'. The same *Guardian* report also featured a study from the Institute of Cancer Research in London which suggested that 'putting off cancer surgeries for three months could lead to almost 5,000 deaths in England alone'.

In July, a report in the *Lancet* concluded that 'substantial increases in the number of avoidable cancer deaths in England are to be expected as a result of diagnostic delays due to the Covid-19 pandemic in the UK.'

Nor were Macmillan and the *Lancet* the only ones to be concerned. An August report in the *Observer* highlighted the huge impact that Covid-19 has had on medical research programmes throughout the UK, noting that 'more than 1,500 clinical trials of new drugs and treatments for cancers, heart disease and other serious illnesses have been permanently closed down in Britain in the wake of the Covid-19 pandemic.'

Meanwhile, cancer charities have been increasingly vocal about the ways in which the funding cuts are affecting them and a leading cancer hospital, the Royal Marsden, recently launched a Covid-19 appeal asking for donations to help 'fund a series of research trials that aim to build on our knowledge of Covid-19 and how the diagnosis, treatment and care of cancer patients can be best managed alongside it'.

Over the past few months, I have heard countless stories of how bad things had become. My oncologist told me that she'd had patients stop treatment because they were terrified of catching the virus and felt they should stay in and self-isolate until the danger had passed. Nurses at my treatment centre talked of a fall in patients – and then once the lockdown eased over the summer of an influx of people presenting with worse symptoms than they might otherwise have had and in considerable pain.

It's here that I have to hold up my hand and admit that the reason my treatment continued uninterrupted was entirely because of my husband, Kris. Not because he made life easier, drove me to appointments and kept both the feral children and our undisciplined dog happy during my lengthy hospital stays (although he did do all of those things), but because he happens to work in a job that comes with private health-care attached.

When the pandemic arrived, it became obvious that receiving my usual treatment at a busy west London hospital would not be possible. They expected to be overrun with Covid patients and were repurposing beds. Cancer patients were advised to avoid coming in if they could possibly do so. At the same time, my treatment was becoming more complicated. Where once my oncologist had envisaged me riding out the pandemic at home with a supply of oral chemo and the odd injection to boost my white blood cells, it was now clear that this would not be possible.

The two main options were to transfer to the Royal Marsden, which meant that I would lose her as an oncologist and have to build a relationship with someone new, or utilise Kris's work-related healthcare and be treated privately. I am very fond of my oncologist, a pragmatic pessimist who has largely kept me sane over the past three years, from the first diagnosis in my breast through to my cancer's sudden spread to the liver, so I chose to stay with her and go private.

I understand that there are some people who will find this decision wrong – and I did struggle with it – but I would say that when you have a disease where the median life expectancy is 11 months after metastasis and you have somehow miraculously made it to 28 months, then you'll pretty much grab at any option that might help you to stay alive.

Even then it wasn't always easy. I have been hospitalised seven times over the course of the past nine months and because of Covid no visitors were allowed to see me, something I found particularly hard during the first admission when I had neutropenic sepsis and acute ascites and spent Easter lying in a bed being given IV antibiotics and blood transfusions.

That experience sharply mirrored those of many cancer patients during the pandemic. While the headlines have, understandably, been all about the awful experiences of those who have had to give birth alone because of Covid, it is hard to describe how very lonely it feels to lie in a hospital bed with only the disease that will kill you for company.

I am not alone in experiencing that loneliness, of course. As the lockdown continued, I spoke both online and on the phone to friends and acquaintances and those who I barely knew about their experiences of the pandemic, the loneliness they felt, the connections they missed, the desire they had simply to go out and talk to other people. They wanted to laugh and cry, drink and dance, to go on holidays, watch films and plays, go to concerts.

I realised, as I lay in my hospital bed, the desire for connection is at its strongest just after it has been taken away. This is what makes so many people dread this new lockdown. The day it was announced, my social media stream was full of people wondering how and if they could really cope with going through it all again.

My own situation remains slightly different. My disease still lives with me, a dark shadow stalking my every move, but it is also the case that it is held in place for now. It is responding to the chemo and thus allowing me to enjoy the ordinary pleasures of our current life: the small joys of opening a new book or discovering a great TV show or singing along loudly to a song you love. The evenings spent laughing uncontrollably with Kris and the kids as they mock me for my dramatic proclamations of imminent death. The visits from friends and family (squeezed in before lockdown) filled with old jokes and new stories and a remembrance of everything we have shared.

Like everyone, there are some things I still miss. Going to the cinema or theatre remains little more than a tantalising dream and I yearn to sit in a Greek taverna watching the sun set or swim in the warming waters of the Mediterranean. Behind those dreams is the ever-present, fear-filled thrum, the beat in your head that says: 'Will I ever do this again? Will life be normal? Or will we forever live in this half-world, remembering the paradise we once had and dreaming of its return?'

So many of those I have spoken to over the past nine months have expressed those fears or similar.

I am not a scientist or an expert in anything and I cannot smile and say that this too will pass. What I am is someone who lives with an ever-present reminder of death and the knowledge that at some point, possibly quite soon, the disease I have will kill me.

It is from the depths of that knowledge that I offer the only piece of advice I can honestly give: even in these depressing times, try to find some part of the day that is worth relishing, whether it is a moment of beauty half-glimpsed outside, the joy found in escaping into a different world on page or screen, or the pleasure of dressing up for yourself and no one else because it makes you feel fine.

The worst thing that you can do is wish your life away thinking of what might have been. Instead, and no matter how hard or how impossible it might seem, try to enjoy at least one moment. None of us, in these most testing of times, know when it might be our last.

The Memory Box

THE MEMORY BOX IS CARVED FROM OAK AND WARDED TO KEEP AWAY BAD SPIRITS. Intricate carvings of apples and ivy cover its lid, alongside rosemary for remembrance. It is the sort of box that wise women and witches once owned and handed down, guarded by spells, filled with love, intended to protect those who own it.

The inside is lined with patches of silk and divided into compartments. In other days and different circumstances, those compartments might have held salt for the preservation of life or herbs to heal and cure. This box is different. This box is not all that it seems.

For a start, look closely and you will see the suggestion that there is another compartment underneath. A private space that can be accessed only by those who know to press the hidden catch and thus release the secrets contained within. This compartment is also bound by spells to ensure that no one can open it except for the two people it is intended for.

But before we get to what it is inside, let us look more closely at the top compartment. It does not, as I have mentioned, contain salt or herbs. Instead, it is filled with dreams. These are the dreams I have caught for my children. My hopes for them when I am gone, for the teenagers they will be and the adults they will grow into. For the love they will find and the careers they will build, the families they may have and the independent lives they will forge without their mother by their side.

Because I am neither a fool nor a hopeless optimist, there is despair here too amid the hope. There will be setbacks. Things will go wrong. Love affairs will falter. Jobs will be lost or struggle to be found. Yet troubles too are part of life and it is in failure and despair as much as in hope and joy that character is formed. We all learn from our mistakes, from those moments when we said too much or not enough, and my children will be no different. I cannot force happiness and success upon them but I can dream of protecting them and of providing them with something to remember me by.

It is for this reason that the top compartment of the memory box contains the letters I have written them. One for each birthday from now until they turn 21, plus a few more to mark special occasions – marriages, births, first jobs, key milestones such as turning 30 and even 40 – those moments when I wish I could be there, holding their hands, laughing with them or putting my arms around them and allowing them to cry.

The chances are that I won't make it through those years, however. That I will not see my children grow up and grow older. I will not watch them finish school or graduate university. I will not dance at their weddings or offer bad advice on how to raise their first child.

It pays to be realistic about this. If you cannot

face death then it is impossible to enjoy life. Similarly, if I cannot acknowledge that I will lose my children then I will never be able to come to terms with the fact that lose them I will, and a good decade earlier than I might I have expected to.

That said, I do not wish to crush them with the weight of expectation or make them feel 'I must do this, it's what my dead mother wanted.' Instead, my biggest dream for both of them is that they are happy in their lives and, more importantly, within themselves. That they grow up to be comfortable in their own skins, eager to express opinions and sure of who they are. I want them to laugh too, long and loud and with their father.

I do not wish for my absence to lie heavy throughout the house that Kris and I created but rather for my presence to feel light, so that when they think of me it is to take the piss, to joke about my worst habits, my tendency to drama, the times I said just the wrong thing and made them all corpse with laughter. I want them to remember the way things were even as they move forward towards the way that they will be.

My children do not have to rule the world (although in my older child Ruby's case, I suspect that she would like to) but simply to enjoy their path through it. To acknowledge that yes, life is sometimes unfair and they were unlucky enough to lose someone they loved and who loved them too. Yes, they may have been marked out as different from other teenagers by that loss, or indeed see themselves as different because of it, but they do not have to be defined by it. Love is always about letting go as much as it is about holding tight and the greatest gift that I can give Ruby and Oisín is the gift of being able to embrace my absence, to remember me always but never to be so oppressed by my death that they cannot move forwards towards the bright, light-filled lives I hope they lead.

If the top compartment of the memory box is filled with dreams and desires for what my children might yet be, the hidden compartment, the one that is for them and them alone, contains my memories, the little moments that I have hugged tight to me since they were born, long before I was diagnosed with a terminal disease.

I see Ruby as a wide-eyed baby staring silently at all around her. As a silent toddler assassin, hanging upside from bookcases, dropping wordlessly from her crib and appearing suddenly, almost shockingly, by my and Kris's side.

I picture her first experience of snow, see her gazing in wonder before bursting out laughing and running down New York's white-covered streets and hear her howls after she shut her fingers in a door moments before the city shut down thanks to the arrival of Hurricane Irene. She is at my friends Rik and Tracy's wedding staring perplexedly at the altar in the distance and saying: 'But, but why is Rik now a little man?'

There is Osh, a fat Russian sailor of a baby, unable to hear because my breast milk is blocking his ear drums, a situation that an excellent ENT specialist will clear up for us after he fails the New York state hearing test three times. He is laughing in his father's arms, smiling at Ruby, who pokes him to see if he will cry.

Older now, he is an escape artist, always looking for the exit sign at every party and running towards it, jumping over barriers, tackling his sister to the ground, an unstoppable, constantly moving force, obsessed with his toy horse Dessie whom he carries with him everywhere. Memorably, just before we leave the city, here he is at a party, holding out a hand to my friend Jane and saying with all the earnestness of a three-year-old: 'Jane, let's dance.'

Fast-forward and we are back in London. They are at nursery and at school and in my parents' back garden playing a ridiculous game which we know as 'Blue Cow', in which I chase them round and round until they collapse heaving with laughter on the ground.

We are in the kitchen mucking around with silly games where I pretend not to understand them and in the small backyard in our rented house in Shepherd's Bush where they paint themselves all over, stick wildflowers in their hair and spend a hot summer's afternoon running around laughing, looking for all the world like a pair of time travellers from a 1970s commune.

We are in Donegal in the woods up the hill from

my parents-in-law's house playing another game called 'Troll Kingdom', where again I chase them, this time through moss-draped trees and over hills. (One day, not too many years later, we will return to Donegal and find the Forestry Commission have cut the trees down, destroying Troll Kingdom. Ruby will be furious, considering it a desecration – arguably her first experience of the power that memories have and the pain you feel when those memories appear ripped away.)

They are growing older, getting more annoyed when things don't work out as planned and winding each other up like a couple of bear cubs. 'It must be so nice to have twins,' a woman says to me. 'We're not twins,' Ruby interjects furiously. 'I'm almost two years older.' And then quietly, so that only I can hear: 'I'm just a bit short.'

Both have a fiercely competitive streak, which Kris, only half-joking, notes they clearly get from me. Thankfully, both of them can let out that burning desire to win by playing sports, from football and basketball to rugby and Gaelic football. Ruby in particular relishes the chance to play the boys at rugby, beating them at their own game. She is competitive at school too, in contrast to her more relaxed brother, determined to be top and irritated when certain subjects prove less easy to her busy mind.

Blink once more and Ruby is a teenager. Experimenting with dress and repeatedly redesigning her room. Shaving off her hair partially in support of me and partially because 'I thought it would look great.' It does.

She is still big eyed and curious about the world, eager to please and desperate to succeed. A talented actress, who won a performing arts scholarship to her state school, she shares my tendency towards the big dramatic gesture, debates passionately, reads voraciously, fidgets constantly and still hangs upside down when we're watching TV. Occasionally she struggles, hating my situation, worrying about her peer group, feeling down about the world. But she is mostly wonderful and when your kids are teens 'mostly' is probably about the best you can achieve.

Oisín is outwardly less complicated. At 11,

almost 12, he is a cheerful, seemingly uncomplicated soul, still prone to curling up for a cuddle or
giving me surprise kisses when I feel tired. Sometimes he lies on my bed next to me and reels off
a list of sporting facts about Tottenham Hotspur.
There is no pressure on me to respond in these
moments; it is enough that I sit there and listen.

Like most boys his age, he spends more time
than he should gaming, although I'm trying hard
to be reasonably relaxed about this, given that he's
talking to friends as he does so. He likes me to play
with him still, computer games, board games and
card games. After years of not reading fiction, he
has discovered Harry Potter and I catch him late at
night still turning 'one last page'. If he thinks about
me dying he never mentions it, preferring spontaneous displays of affection over attempts to talk.

Do I worry about this? Of course. I worry that,
like his father, he is the sort of person who may
keep all his feelings locked inside. That he won't
speak of grief or loss or death or dying until one
day the tsunami of loss overwhelms him. Then I
watch him horsing around with the dog, cuddling

him, walking him night after night and I think he'll be fine. When he needs to, he will talk. Until then, why ruin the uncomplicated pleasures of being a largely uncomplicated age?

Their memories are here too. It is important that they do not see me as Saint Mum, the dead angel in heaven, but rather that they remember me in all my imperfections. Throwing shoes, shouting, losing my temper at just the wrong moment. Loving them fiercely too, reading to them, checking their homework, making sure that, despite everything, they feel wanted and adored.

I joke sometimes that in the future, when they feel the wind howling and rain pouring and a storm threatening to break then it will be me stomping around having a quick temper tantrum. When the weather breaks and the sun starts to shine then it will be a sign that I've calmed down. It's a silly joke but one that makes them laugh, as they laugh too when they misbehave and I frown and say be careful or when I'm dead I'll haunt you and check that you're not messing Dad around and acting the fool.

These then are my memories. So many of them

that they threaten to spill out from the box, float-ing off into the world, more vivid to me than a photograph, vital moments imprinted on my brain.

They are, of course, intensely personal. I share them not, I hope, through self-indulgence but because I think that when death starts to lurk around every corner so the moments you once had become ever more vivid and intensely real.

They are my gift to my children and to Kris. In the same way that this book is, too. For what I want to say to them most of all, after everything has been written down, everything shared, is that while death might be inevitable and yes, it is better in many ways if you are prepared, for you, my children, it is hopefully many years away. Until then, I want you to live, to love, to find enjoyment where you can and to understand that loss is sim-ply a small part of a greater human experience. It is that refrain that I whisper as I stand outside your doors each night: make the most of your life, live to the fullest and worry about what will hap-pen after, when and if it comes.

Endnote
by Kristian Glynn

I HAVE GIVEN MYSELF QUITE THE CHALLENGE HERE. Sitting down the day after our son Oisín's twelfth birthday, attempting to put into words what I want to say about Sarah and the pressure of having them sit beside her accomplished, clever and funny writing is not a task I found myself jumping into lightly. How to sum up a person in just a few thousand words who meant so much to so many? How to do justice to the person my world revolved around? It's another task that demonstrates my, our, loss. It's another thing that would work a lot better if Sarah were here to smooth the rough edges. If she could be here to gently suggest changes and generally fix everything, as she always did for family who had to commit words to paper. I should say at this point that my outlook is to want to celebrate the time we had together and be thankful for that, rather than be sad for what we have lost.

One of the things that has been brought into sharp focus since her death is that when people use the term 'other half' it really means exactly what it says: the other half of every conversation you want to have is missing; the other half of your bed is empty every morning and every night; there is a hole in the other half of every single event in your children's lives. I won't be able to adequately articulate how much and in how many uncountable ways I miss her. I even miss the many hospital trips because it was time spent together talking about anything and everything. Everything seems to remind me of Sarah. Our house, which is pretty much a monument to books, food (including the obligatory big table) and the artwork and pictures she carefully selected, has her touch everywhere and that brings me comfort, even down to the rigorous book order I'll never be able to replicate or add to. There is too much to say about Sarah to fully do her justice so, with no apologies, I am going to skip over most of the illness as that has been well covered. I want to share the Sarah that I knew, and the life we had together.

Sarah and I were friends for years before we finally got together. We shared a love for National Hunt racing (it is no coincidence our firstborn is called Ruby) and Tottenham Hotspur – though they loved us back in varying degrees – and when we finally did get together we wasted no time. We were pretty much inseparable. We got married, moved to New York and had our first child in quick succession. We didn't take life particularly seriously and it's fair to say both of us were terrible with money (or pretty good with it, depending on your outlook). This, coupled with a taste for the finer things in life, meant we crammed in a lot of fun without a single regret. She loved a live event, be it racing, football, a concert or a book launch, and the excitement and energy of the experience was always a worthwhile one. Now (and over the last few years), I have begun doing this with the children: in the last few days alone we attended a Kano concert and saw the mighty Tottenham Hotspur confound many by beating the media darlings and champions, who are in no way part of the ruining of football with their petrodollars, Manchester City. She would have loved both.

She was gorgeous, clever and funny and brought with her a wonderful family and a wide circle of friends, who I am very thankful for. She was amazingly well read and knowledgeable with a wicked sense of humour and an occasionally filthy laugh. She had no time for book or TV snobbery – she adored Jilly Cooper but was as equally at home with *Crime and Punishment* (which she read on our honeymoon in St Petersburg and Moscow as part of a specially curated list of Russia-related books).

We settled into New York life easily. Sarah loved New York and always said it was the city of her soul. Her easy, empathetic nature meant that she made lots of interesting friends as she and baby Ruby traversed the streets and coffee shops of Brooklyn. One thing I always marvelled at was her ability to maintain such long-standing friendships, given her rudimentary technological abilities and aversion to taking down details. But somehow she was in touch with people from all periods of her life. This became abundantly clear to me after her death and I was blown away by all the tributes that she received. I was also thrilled she had inspired such followings online through her work.

In case it wasn't already clear, Sarah was one of the lucky few who really loved her job. So much so that, even in her last days, filing copy was near the top of her priority list. Doctors, specialists, nurses (and me as well, to be fair to the brilliant staff) were all shooed away at various points with the words 'I'm on deadline'. They also got short shrift in the most important week in March as 'the racing's on'. Without wanting to dwell on this time, it is these attributes and that focus that made her so brilliant. Nothing was going to distract from the good things, from the writing and the racing and friends and family. Not even the grind of her treatment. Plus, alongside me and the children, she had our errant but adored dog Murphy, who we got just before she was diagnosed, to keep her busy.

While she wrote for many papers, she was at heart an '*Observer* person'. When we first started seeing each other, she was working there and she was thrilled to be 'banged out' of the newsroom, a true journalist's farewell, when she left to move to America. No Sunday was complete without the whole suite of papers bought and, as the day went on, discarded on the floor, section by section. She believed so wholeheartedly in her trade and it being as important if not more so than it has ever been. Her willingness to write about difficult topics in her own life as they may help others only made me more proud of her, and all the tributes she received for her work, throughout her career, made me hope that she had some sense of how well regarded she was professionally. I think her great empathy made her the writer she was. She had such a strong sense of injustice and an ear for anyone's story, which maybe explains the strength of her personal relationships.

I also think what made her work so well received was that when she liked something she was unashamed in wholeheartedly going into bat for it. This came out in every facet of her life. Rarely did someone leave our house without a book or TV recommendation (or, in many cases, without an actual book). That's what she was like about everything: she was fiercely passionate with strong opinions and that was one of the many things I loved about her.

A good example is her questionable gambling strategy of 'have a strong opinion and dive right in'. As previously noted, our profligacy and wayward tendencies were well matched, but in the grand scheme of things, we were in the grey if not black, rather than the red. A favourite memory, and great example of this, comes from back in late 2005 or early 2006. I woke up at around 3am with a tenuous theory as to why War of Attrition was going to win the Cheltenham Gold Cup. I realised I had to wake Sarah and tell her in case

I forgot this theory. Instead of the expletives that could have come it was duly noted and on the day, when the gates opened, she strode up to the bookie with the best odds to stick £50 on the nose. We had gone to Cheltenham with the grandiose plan of winning the money for our engagement ring – a ruby, of course – which we achieved. But the moment when Conor O'Dwyer crossed the finish line on War of Attrition was the one time in my life I can truly say it was like being in a movie. It felt like the crowds parted as we hugged and jumped for joy, before quickly turning our attention to the foxhunters.

In 2009, Oisín was born and somehow she managed to balance both children and her freelance career without that much fuss. We muddled along not really doing anything by the book but those years in New York were probably the happiest of our lives. While we missed family and friends, we had a steady stream of visitors from home and lots of good friends in the city. One of Sarah's hallmarks was an ability to throw together an amazing dinner at the drop of a hat. On occasion, this could be for large numbers – as she said in an earlier chapter, she loved to have a big crowd round a table with no topic off limits for discussion.

Today, when I look at the children, they exhibit many of the characteristics that made her the brilliant person she was. She never talked down to them and that is clear in their personalities. They are articulate, fiercely loyal, empathetic and caring. They are a constant inspiration to me. Her unique parenting style may have raised the occasional eyebrow: not many kids get sung to sleep with the Irish rebel song 'Kevin Barry' and it's rare to see a three-year-old being read Edward Gorey's *Gashlycrumb Tinies* on the subway.

She also loved to travel and we had many memorable holidays as a family: going back to New York after our return to England, various Greek islands, New Orleans and Jamaica. We were also lucky enough to have an occasional getaway together – often to Paris, on *Prix de L'arc de Triomphe* weekend. Our weekends away would invariably be spent reading, eating and drinking, and only occasionally speaking, as we were at such ease in our own little world. Every city break would contain a trudge to a bookshop where Sarah could be found sat in a corner with a mountain of books to whittle down to a more manageable pile to purchase. No visit to Dublin could start without a trip to Hodges Figgis, nor a trip to Paris without dropping by Shakespeare and Co. Sarah even managed to find the English language bookshops in Moscow while on our honeymoon (a more successful outing than trying to purchase a pregnancy test kit from an increasingly bemused shop assistant near Red Square).

Our family holidays provide some of the fondest memories. There is many a hotel that has been enriched by a bunch of her discarded holiday books, yet she still found ample time to play in the pool or on the beach with the kids. Sarah loved the coast and occasionally we would drive out on a whim just to see the sea and blow the cobwebs away. Our last holiday to Jamaica was particularly idyllic as we swam in the stunning, warm ocean and enjoyed such memorable and wonderful hospitality.

At this point, it would be remiss not to highlight the amazing support, help and generosity we received from friends and family over the years. I could never thank people enough.

In some ways, there was a certain liberation for Sarah in knowing her cancer was going to kill her. She didn't suddenly become a health obsessive – it didn't change her in that respect – but she also didn't waste any time on things that weren't worth it. She didn't have time for regrets, either. She enjoyed her life and her work, and her passion and determination shone through. She had fierce love for her family and for her friends.

Sarah's attitude allowed us to discuss the future and how life would have to go on. The hopes and dreams she had for the children live on; she was so proud of them, they were the centre of her world. When she was first diagnosed, her thoughts were not of herself but for us, her family, and that focus tells you all you need to know about her.

Covid robbed her of lots of things, like it did many others. She longed to spend as much time as possible with her family and friends; she longed for beach holidays and restaurants (which she made up for with a production line of expensive meal kits). Though sometimes confined to her hospital bed alone and without visitors, she refused to let cancer define or defeat her, and this determination enabled her to come home and die peacefully, just as she wanted, with the help of her wonderful goddaughter Sefi, without whom it wouldn't have been possible.

Despite all the restrictions, we gave her the send-off she described in the first chapter. She had magnificent black-plumed horses who stopped traffic all the way from the abbey to the cemetery. We held the beautiful ceremony, the chorister playing 'On Raglan Road', a reading from Louis MacNeice, and she was played out to 'Carrickfergus'. While we could only have 30 people at the service, many of her friends were with us watching online or outside the church to see her off. It wasn't a maudlin affair; there was a lot of joy and laughter, the way she had planned it.

Today, our lives have a massive gulf in them and every piece of happiness or happy occasion has a tint of sadness. I hope that subsides eventually. We have had a lots of firsts to get through – holidays, birthdays, anniversaries and so on – but she wouldn't have much time for anything more melancholy than that.

One of Sarah's key pieces of advice was to never be the last to leave a party and while she is right about that, I just wish she could have stuck around and had another couple for the road.